A. J. Culyer

Measuring Health:
lessons for Ontario

PUBLISHED FOR THE ONTARIO ECONOMIC COUNCIL BY
UNIVERSITY OF TORONTO PRESS
TORONTO   BUFFALO   LONDON

© Ontario Economic Council 1978
Reprinted 2015
ISBN 978-0-8020-3354-3 (paper)

Canadian Cataloguing in Publication Data

Culyer, A.J., 1942-
  Measuring health

  (Ontario Economic Council research studies; 14
  ISSN 0078-5091)

  Bibliography: p.
  ISBN 978-0-8020-3354-3 (pbk.)

  1. Medical care — Evaluation. 2. Medical care —
  Ontario — Evaluation. I. Title. II. Series: Ontario
  Economic Council. Ontario Economic Council research
  studies; 14.

  RA395.C2C85   362.1'09713   C77-001553-0

This study reflects the views of the author and not necessarily those
of the Ontario Economic Council.

Contents

Acknowledgments

My principal thanks must go to the Ontario Economic Council whose chairman, Grant Reuber, and past and present research directors, Colin Hindle and Don Dawson, have done so much to make my all-too-brief stay both pleasant and productive. Second, I owe an inestimable debt to the research staff of the Council for their instructive comments on my work, both formal and informal. In particular, Pran Manga not only gave me useful insights into the Ontario health system of which his knowledge is immense, but also gave freely and willingly of his time when I needed a testing ground on which to try some ideas. His successor, Morris Barer, has also proved to be a constructive but kind critic.

George Torrance and Alan Wolfson, at McMaster and the University of Toronto respectively, are two people who are not only kind beyond measure and have been of immense help to me, but who simply must be mentioned by virtue of the fact that I have shamelessly plundered their best ideas. I hope they can still recognize them.

Dan Markovich, whose painstaking research is particularly worthy of admiration in chapter seven, not only obtained all the data I wanted by the time I needed them but managed to do so and still serve the insatiable statistical appetite of Robin Milne. I have also learned much, and got fewer things wrong than otherwise would have been the case, as a result of seminars at the OEC, the Economics Departments at the universities of Guelph and Trent, the Economics Department and the School of Social Work, both at McMaster University, and the Institute for Policy Analysis and the Department of Health Administration, both at the University of Toronto.

Finally, and by no means least, my thanks for the patience with which the administrative, library, and secretarial staff at the OEC coped with my excessive demands on their time. To Paul Lonergan, who keeps the office in first-rate running order, and to Carol, Chris, Hilda, June, Kathy, and Mary, my heartfelt appreciation.

MEASURING HEALTH: LESSONS FOR ONTARIO

1
Introduction

'The good health of Canadians is an objective that shines brightly above the thicket of jurisdictions and special interest groups.' (Lalonde, 1974, 66). That noble sentiment can readily be found expressed, though often with less euphony, in the utterances of federal and provincial ministers, in the ramblings of royal commissions, in the constitution of the World Health Organization, in the introductory lectures of professors of public health and of clinical medicine, in the Hippocratic oath. Although there is dispute about the extent to which the value embodied in this assertion conflicts with others, such as individual freedom or the residuum of the 'less eligibility' principles inherited by North America from the Elizabethan Poor Law, its *empirical* content – the measurement of health or ill-health – is the central topic of this book. It is certainly central to the 'three Es' of health care: effectiveness, efficiency, and equity. The meaning, relevance, and measurability of this central triad are our concern throughout the following chapters, as are the value questions to which they give rise.

Although the conceptual framework in terms of which we shall discuss the 'three Es' is that of the economist, it is a matter about which we are unrepentant, partly because the conceptions offered by economics are useful tools and partly because using this framework will give us an opportunity to emphasize that economics is not a mere method of cash accounting but is concerned at its root and foundation with precisely the 'three Es' which we are concerned with here.

The Canadian economist Robert Evans, in a brilliantly perspicacious review of a recent health economics conference (Evans, 1976) identifies two types of health economist: N (narrow) and B (board). The Ns (mostly American) believe that the consumer sovereignty economic model, with its traditional supply-demand framework and assumption of efficient markets, is an appropriate basis both for empirical studies of health services and for evaluative appraisal. The Bs (rest of the world, including Canada) find these assumptions, both in empirical and evaluative work, unrealistic and unhelpful. They emphasize, in particular, the crucial role of physicians in regulating supply and demand, and the fact that the social interest in health care is a good deal more than merely the sum of individual consumer's *private* demands for health or medical care.

The present work is written by a member of the 'rest of world' team. For this reason, the reader will find here considerably more discussion of the 'philosophical' (though this is, perhaps, too pretentious an adjective) underpinnings of the health measurement literature. In this book it is argued that the objective of the provincial health care system ought to be – even though it may not always appear actually to be – the province's health and *not* the maximization of consumers' (or producers') satisfactions. We shall also, however, attempt to show that our approach does not require us to jettison entirely the individualistic philosophical foundations of contemporary economics. What instead we have to do is to recognize that ill-health is not merely the private matter the N-types take it to be. Nor is it, as governments appear sometimes to believe, mainly of concern because it reduces GNP, or increases transfer payments. Ill-health is not an 'indirect' cost of sickness, to be weighed in the balance somehow, and in unquantified form, with the dollars spent and gained in attempts to reduce it. With such a perception, the dollars will always triumph over the dolours. Whether we like it or not, the active participation of the state in planning and running health services is here to stay. What we have to do is to guard against the evident danger that the earlier injustices of the unassisted market are not replaced by a new philistinism in which the government reduces the problems of health care planning to a series of crude business stratagems.

If the claims made by cost-benefit enthusiasts are sometimes pretentious and promise far more than they can ever deliver, there is little doubt in my own mind that the approach they advocate is basically sound. But the cause will not be won by extravagant claims and know-all criticism of what presently goes on. There is only one way, and that is by persuasion: by *persuading* decision-makers that there does exist expertise in measuring dimensions of ill-health, defined in terms of individuals' ability to function, that can be brought into the decisionmaking framework and that can help clarify objectives, help assess the extent of their attainment and help evaluate alternative means of doing so.

I do not believe that it would be either prudent or sensible to design, at least in the foreseeable future, a blue-print for planning health care in Ontario on the basis of health measurement. Present techniques are too crude for that.

Moreover, they are also new and have yet to win acceptance by planners and practitioners alike. The time is ripe, however, for the knowledge and experience which has to date been built up to be communicated to a wider audience, including planners and practitioners. The time is also ripe for the basic statistical information to be gathered. It is to assist in this wider dialogue and to outline the features of the desirable statistics that the present work has its principal justification. The literature of health measurement is distributed far and wide in technical papers and monographs written by persons from a dozen disciplinary backgrounds and methodologies. I have attempted to bring this work together and, for the first time, to attempt a comprehensive review; not papering over the cracks, nor poking a pocket knife into every piece of suspect woodwork, but investigating the soundness of the basic structure and showing how it has proved to have load-bearing strengths.

For illustration I have drawn, where possible, on local sources. It is fortunate that some of the most effective pioneering work in this territory has taken place here in Ontario, notably by George Torrance at McMaster University and Alan Wolfson at the University of Toronto. In one or two small ways I have extended their work in order to paint a more detailed or up-to-date picture. I make no claim, however, to any extensive original empirical work. In addition to the work which has used Ontarian data in the context of Ontarian institutions, I have also tried to identify some decision-making areas in Ontario where there seems to be a demand for some of the techniques described here. It would be imprudent for a visiting foreign scholar to attempt to prescribe, on the basis of a nine-month sojourn, where and how health measurement should be used in Ontario, particularly since much of his time has been behind a desk trying to grapple with the extensive and multi-disciplinary literature. But I have become aware, from conversations with many who are concerned, both directly and indirectly, with evaluative analysis of the provincial health services, that there exists substantial potential for the application of the techniques to be described. To my mind, there exists an overwhelming case for the establishment of several pools of (multi-disciplinary) expertise in evaluation, using health measurement techniques, at provincial centres. Such pools should both develop a research programme of substantial size and be available as technical resources both to the local and the wider provincial communities. The new division of community health in the Faculty of Medicine at the University of Toronto which combines behavioural science, epidemiology, biostatistics, and health administration may be one natural location of such a group. Potential clients of such groups would range from those engaged in clinical research into the effects of interventions on the natural history of disease, or economic research into the cost-effectiveness of alternative regimes of care, through members of District Health Councils in need of monitoring the performance of the health services in their areas, to provincial level concern in, for example, the Ministry of Health or the Royal Colleges, with devising allocation criteria, ensuring accessibility, or monitoring the quality of care.

The more one reflects upon it, however, the more it is clear that Ontario, though fortunate in having both some pioneers in our territory and a record system in OHIP that lends itself to particular kinds of measure not easily available elsewhere, is far from unique in the problems it faces at root level. Although the administrative structure is different both from other Canadian provinces and other countries, the basic concerns embodied in the 'three Es' and the basic information that is needed to reach satisfactory solutions are, in all essential features, the same. The most basic of all the information that is needed relates to the health status of individuals and populations and that remains true in the highly pluralistic system of the USA, the unitary system of the UK, and in the constitutionally provincial system of Canada.

It is the increasing awareness of our need for such basic information as well as an awareness that existing measures of life expectancy, mortality and morbidity do not provide it, that has given impetus to the health measurement research program, a program that has developed so far that few planners or practitioners will have had much opportunity, even if they had the ability, to keep up with developments. The first need, then, is for the potential clients to be brought up to date concerning what is possible, how what is possible can be used and what its shortcomings are. Responsible and highly-trained professional men and women in the health services cannot be expected to accept, let alone to use, what they do not understand or what they are gravely suspicious of. Unfortunately, there exists at present no 'manual,' no 'guide,' no really comprehensive assessment of the health measurement literature that is accessible to those outside the ranks of the researching in-group. In attempting to provide an initiation that is comprehensive, painless, and persuasive, it has not proved possible (at least for this author) to avoid all technicalities. Most of them are in chapter five, which may be skimmed over by those who find them daunting or whose chief interest lies in their application. There is also, I fear, much unnecessary jargon which has persisted despite my attempts to purge the text. I hope that where I have fallen victim to the inelegancies of my own discipline's vocabulary, I shall be forgiven by those whose inelegancies derive from other sources and that I shall not, through my own infelicity of expression, do disservice to the cause which we all in the end are trying to serve.

I hope also, however, to have provided more than merely a methodological review, literature assessment, and 'state of the art' report. In particular, I would hope that two other worthy causes had also been promoted. The first is to persuade *economists,* including most health economists, and including those employed in the ministries and organizations responsible for health care delivery, that they should take far more seriously than is their wont both the language of 'need' so beloved by many other social scientists and the conceptual developments that have been reported in Operations Research and medical journals and monographs, whose contents most of them would not even think to scan. Economists are not without influence and much of what follows is designed to show that ideas that appear to be alien to economics turn out, on closer inspection, not to be so alien after all. When they happen to be good ideas as well, economists should readily absorb them into the corpus of their thought. The second worthy cause brings us back to Marc Lalonde.

If 'the good health of Canadians is an objective that shines brightly above the thicket of jurisdictions and special interest groups' it is surely time that we attempted seriously to apply some of the good ideas that exist about how the objective may be measured. *A New Perspective on the Health of Canadians* (1974) was quite explicit about it: 'What is really needed is a measure of the prevalence of ill-health in the population, counting not only mortality and hospital morbidity, but illness treated by health professionals outside hospital, illnesses which are self-treated or self-limiting, undetected morbidity, and a count of the chronically disabled' (pp. 23-4). The best way of doing this is by measuring *health status* itself. The following chapters try to show what might be done, both at the macrocosmic level envisaged by the Lalonde document and the Canada Health Survey and at more microcosmic levels, and what problems of concept and of value must be solved if the noble sentiment of our opening quotation is to be an (approximately) operational objective.

It is worth adding that research in Canada – in particular the development of the Canada Health Survey and Canada's co-operation in OECD work in the health indicators field – is ongoing. Accordingly, when at various points in the book we have discussed – and sometimes been critical of – recent developments, such discussion is intended to be a helpful input into the ongoing dialogue. Such is the pace at which work is progressing, and such are the lags in the production of books that in some details the discussion here may have been overtaken by events (see, for example, Romeder and Hill, 1977).

A final word is due concerning the order of the argument in this book. Unlike reading a thriller, it helps here to know the dénouement when one is still at the beginning. Since chapter eight provides both a summary of the main points in each chapter and the principal recommendations made for Ontario policy, it would probably be best read before chapter two. The remaining chapters are ordered in the way that makes, I trust, the best logical sense.

2
Indicators and indexes:
an overview

Interest in health measurement has tended to concentrate around two focal points which have come to be associated with the terms 'indicator' and 'index'. The former tend to refer to rather aggregate measures intended for use as complements to GNP data and the latter tend to refer to more microcosmic measures of use in clinical practice or the cost-effectiveness of alternative regimes of care. Historically, in the health territory (as in other territories), these two views have developed more or less independently of one another. Yet the basic problems confronted by each are actually the same (as we shall see later in chapters four and five) and insights are to be gained from seeing both as special cases of a more general measurement problem.

SOCIAL INDICATORS OF HEALTH

(a) *Indicators in general*
A natural starting point for any discussion of social indicators in Canada is contained in the eighth, eleventh, and twelfth annual reviews of the Economic Council of Canada (Economic Council of Canada, 1971, 1974, and 1975) and the detailed rationale of indicators written for the ECC by Henderson (Henderson, 1974). The ECC recommended the 'development of a comprehensive set of statistical measures to monitor the changing conditions of our society over a broad spectrum of concerns' (ECC, 1971, 70-1). A similar general motive lies behind the social indicator programme of the OECD. As its Council of Economic Ministers has said: 'growth is not an end in itself, but rather an instrument for creating better conditions of life ... increased attention must be

given to the qualitative aspects of growth, and to the formulation of policies with respect to the broad economic and social choices involved in the allocation of growing resources' (OECD, 1976).[1]

Similar arguments have been put for the USA and UK. Olson (1969) writes for the USA: 'for all their virtues, the national income statistics don't tell us what we need to know about the condition of American society. They leave out the learning of our children, the quality of our culture, the advance of science, the compatability of our families, the liberties and democratic processes we cherish. They neglect the pollution of the environment, the degradations [sic] of crime, and the toll of sickness' (86). In Britain the focus has been placed more firmly on policy relevance than is frequently found: 'the objective of *Social Trends* remains that of presenting a manageable set of statistical series relating to social policies and conditions which will provide a picture of some significant ways in which our society is changing. This means giving information about people, rather than about government or institutions ... The selection aims primarily at providing a source of background data for policy makers and administrators ... in the hope that this provides pointers to tomorrow's problems while showing the combined effects of today's solutions' (CSO, 1975, 8, 9).

Common to all of these endeavours seem to be the following two objectives: (i) to provide measures (or methods of getting measures) that fill in gaps in knowledge about socio-economic conditions: (ii) to reduce information overload by eliminating measures that are redundant either by virtue of their policy irrelevance or because they merely duplicate information given by other measures (OECD, 1976, 5). But other objectives seem also to be present from time to time. One of these consists in the development of empirical counterparts to one or another general model or theory of the social system. The verdict on this aspiration has characteristically been adverse. For example, Henderson at

---

1 Additional reports to those mentioned in the text are: *Perspective Canada* (Ottawa, Statistics Canada, 1974); *Données sociales* (Paris, INSEE, 1973); *Gesellschaftlichen Daten 1973* (Bonn: Bundesministerium fur Arbeit Socialordnung, 1973); *The Life and its Quality in Japan* (Tokyo: Economic Planning Agency, 1973); *Social Indicators of Japan* (Tokyo: Research Committee of the Council of National Living, 1974); *Sociaal en Cultureel Rapport 1974* (The Hague: Social and Cultural Planning Bureau, 1974); *Socialt Utsyn* (Oslo: Central Statistical Bureau, 1974); *Panoramica Social* (Madrid: National Statistical Institute, 1975); *Levnadsforhallenden Arsbok 1975* (Stockholm: National Central Bureau of Statistics, 1975); *Economic Report 1974-1975* (Kuala Lumpur: Treasury, 1973); *Socioeconomic Indicators and National Policy* (Kuala Lumpur: Department of Statistics, 1974); *Measuring the Quality of Life: Phillippines Social Indicators* (Tagaytay City: Development Academy of the Phillippines, 1975). I have not had the opportunity to study most of these.

the beginning of his book, says: 'though there are a number of approaches to conceptualizing a general social system theory, none of these has yet been developed to a level that would permit a simultaneous comprehensive examination of the impact of particular activities on all facets of all social system. Such a model – which would make possible a form of "social accounting" – cannot even be said to be on the horizon, in any practical sense' (Henderson, 1974, 7). The danger of a too ready dismissal of this possibility is, however, apparent: absence of such a general theory leads to the (false) inference that no general principles at all can be applied, with the result that social indicator development degenerates into an orgy of *ad hoc* measurement of *ad hoc* entities as determined by some unstructured (and also *ad hoc*) politico-administrative bargaining procedure. Moreover, it is the firm view taken here that a general theory – albeit of a particular kind – is not in fact unavailable and so the rejection of its implications is unnecessary as well as dangerous.

What does seem to be absent is the kind of *general* sociological theory of society discussed in Parsons *et al.* (1961) to which the social indicators literature makes frequent reference. Some would doubt whether the development of a truly general theory of this sort makes any kind of scientific sense at all. Be that as it may, there are certainly other kinds of theory which claim to relate to specific and measurable entities which are of policy – and not merely academic – concern. One set of such theories, which need not detain us long in view of their familiarity, is provided by the economics of aggregate social indicators in macroeconomic models. But there is also a wealth of other possible sources for theoretical underpinning. For example, there are sociological, epidemiological, etiological, demographic, and economic theories of disease and ill-health and of effective and efficient decision-making in the health services which have most of the features usually associated with a general theory of social indicators. Thus there are theories – some of them well-tested and widely agreed – of the interaction of various environmental, demographic, housing, nutritional, and health service variables with etiological factors in desease. There are theories which relate the use of *resources* in one area (e.g., health) with their use in another (e.g., education) via their effectiveness, cost, location, etc. What is true of health is true also of many other specific areas of potential interest.

A characteristic of much of this theorizing is its non-normative or positive nature. It does not aim to prescribe or recommend – to tell society how it should chose. What it does do is to explain what is likely to happen to one variable, or set of variables, as another variable or set of variables alters or is altered. The kind of general model of which the above are examples is, of course, quite obviously a model well suited to the purpose of aiding decision-makers to make decisions. Indeed, typically these theories have been evolved for precisely that purpose.

Related to these, however, is a set of *normative* theories whose relevance is to organize the positive theories in order that value inferences may be drawn. Characteristic of such theories are ethical notions of justice, economic notions of efficiency or political notions of expediency. The questions to which these theories address themselves concern the ends (or objectives) of policy and the 'best' means of attaining those ends.

This perspective on a model of social indicators has been succinctly put in the OECD program: 'If the overall objective of policies is to improve social well-being, that concept must first be made operational: goal areas must be defined and expressed in such a way that changes in them can be monitored. Next, the concept of well-being needs to be related to the various factors by which it is influenced and these variables, as well as their relative impact, must be monitored. Thirdly, the relative impact of policy measures on these influencing factors needs to be ascertained. Lastly, the use of resources in existing and alternative policy measures should be monitored' (OECD, 1976, 5).

The spirit of this quotation is plainly similar to that of the British CSO quoted above (p. 9): focus is to be upon those social phenomena which can be affected by policy instruments. From this we are led directly into the following broad tripartite classification of social indicators: indicators of output or outcome; indicators of *value* of output; and indicators of the relationship between inputs and output. In the health territory, these were described as measures of the state-of-Health, measures of the need-for-Health and measures of the effectiveness of health-affecting activities by Culyer, Lavers, and Williams (1971, 31).

The evidently instrumental nature of this view of social indicators, with its clear distinction of principle between ends and means and its analytic setting firmly based on a decision-theoretic foundation, owes a great deal to economic theory and to the work of economists in developing both conceptual and empirical aspects of social indicators. The rationale has been clearly put by the present author and his colleagues:

Need indicators are required in order to establish priorities. Not all needs can be met and some are more urgent than others. Essentially, a Need indicator would have to combine two elements: a social and humanitarian value upon an improvement in the community's health and the value of the other socially and compassionately desired programmes that would have to be gone without as a result of devoting more resources to health.

Effectiveness indicators are required in order to achieve an objective stated in terms of the State indicator. Thus, one use for the Effectiveness indicator would be to demonstrate how by varying one such input the State indicator would respond during various time periods, or to show how different inputs may substitute for one another in promoting a given State or change of State.

Essentially Effectiveness indicators provide the technical relationships between inputs and outputs. We do not underestimate the practical problems of discovering these relationships with an degree of precision.

Obviously, however, logically prior to both Need and Effectiveness indicators is the State indicator, since both of the former are variables – in principle one socially decided, the other technically determined – expressed as a function of the State indicator. If the problem of the State indicator cannot be solved, or what is a very similar thing, the problem of *output* of health services, then no progress will be possible with the other two, for the objectives of policy, we believe, ought ultimately to be definable in terms of the state of the community's health. (Culyer, Lavers, and Williams, 1971, 8-9)

The decision-theory/problem-solving nature of this approach can easily be defended on pragmatic grounds, for the chief factor leading to the elaboration of social indicators research programmes has undoubtedly been the increasing scale on which governments have sought to control and monitor the life of society. Advances in economics in the 1930s and 1940s gave a new shape to the kind of governmental intervention in the control of the economy (and not merely in the aggregate) in response to widely-expressed dissatisfaction with the way in which it was working. The fact that governments have increasingly been unable to resist further extensions of their activity into the 'social' territory is scarcely, however, attributable to the influence of social theorists. The actual reasons are not our concern here, but what is quite clear is that in a society where an individual's 'welfare' would be determined only by his own choices and where it is largely regarded as his own business only, the kind of data collected as social indicators would have little value. The situation is quite the contrary where neither of these assumptions holds and this, of course, is generally the case. Unless the state is to be permitted to become (continue to be?) an irrational leviathan thrashing around in a sea of expanding obligations but with diminishing ability either to monitor or control the way it meets them, the informational needs served by social indicators having the kind of decision-making rationale here described become an increasingly important part of the functioning of the state.

There are, of course, alternative views. Some, for example, find the whole business to be an unfortunate attempt to prolong the life of a leviathan whose early demise is most earnestly to be welcomed. For them the leviathan's thrashing around is hopefully the onset of its death throes. To the extent that this reaction is in the head rather than the gut the answer is clear: the model of social indicators developed here does *not* assume that the social aims of society (however these may be determined) are necessarily best served by the direct instrumentality of the state. If 'society' (which we shall have to define) cares about the education and health (whatever these may mean) of its children then there is no presumption that any one *means* of effecting certain ends in education and health is to be preferred. Indeed it is precisely in order to enable a more rational selection from among competing ends and competing means of achieving any one end that the social indicators research program exists.

Another school deplores the hard means-ends approach embodied in the paradigm. 'The end can never justify the means' is the familiar battle-cry of this school. To the extent that this reaction is in the head rather than the heart the answer is again clear: if the ends cannot justify the means then certainly nothing else can. This is not to say that some end will justify all or any means, but it is to assert that means are not the same as ends, that ends can and do conflict and that not all means are equally functional at meeting a given bundle of ends.

A third school will argue that it is illusion to suppose that the social ills which beset society can be mitigated by the tinkering, Fabian approach apparently implicit in the social indicators framework. We would probably be wise to acknowledge the possibility that this school of thought may be correct. It may be that the underlying roots of social problems cannot be severed without fundamental change in society and social indicators are therefore of limited usefulness. It may be, we should acknowledge, that advanced capitalism is ineradicably blighted. However, having acknowledged that this *may* be true, we do not have to suppose that it actually *is*. The evidence that the known alternatives to capitalism deliver a total bundle of social characteristics that people manifestly prefer is thin to vanishing point. Moreover – and this is more deplorable even than the poverty of the evidence – we simply do not have a sufficiently well-articulated theory of the relationship between the institutions of modern capitalism and social problems that has logical appeal (quite aside from empirical validity) of an obviously greater degree than the kind of models upon which the social indicator program is, explicitly and implicitly, built. At the very least, we might hope that the international comparisons of social indicators might shed light on the more grandiloquent issues involved in the choice of social system. These critics, then, make an act of faith. They may be right. But their act is very much a blind one and by making it they deny the desirability of trying to adduce some evidence that may have a bearing on the point.

A related objection, often coming from the same school, concerns the alleged total inadequacy of the description of the objectives of society, as well as the mis-specification of the causes of and means of affecting social outcomes. According to this most fundamentally radical view of all, the West burns while bourgeois social scientists fiddle. In this view, the problems of society are the outcome of the socializing institutions of capitalist society (family, advertising, schools, universities and, above all, capitalist and state-capitalist productive enterprises) which cause individuals to be 'alienated from themselves' as self-development and preference or value formation are conditioned to conform to the requirements of the capitalist order. 'Alienation' then becomes the core of social problems and is one of the inevitable contradictions of the capitalist order. Social indicators as they seem to be developing would, in this version of the radical view, be seen essentially as a sentimental framework for measuring largely irrelevant phenomena and talking about them in a largely irrelevant way — *a fortiori* if the indicators are designed for a client that is the bourgeois state itself.

The extreme radical view is much like the curate's egg. The good part consists in its warning that our whole analysis of indicators must be shot through with values whose sources and embodiments should never be taken for granted but subject to continuing scrutiny and questioning. As we shall see later, these values are not merely to do with the more ultimate ends of society but permeate the idea of social measurement throughout — in our special case they permeate, for example, the whole concept of 'health' measurement itself. Fortunately, when the analysis comes down from the level of high generality to specifics, the question of values also becomes more specific and, we believe, discussable in a fruitful way. The existence of values in the analysis is, of course, inescapable. What is to be escaped is the assertion of any particular set of values *a priori* or the implicit infiltration of any set from a currently dominant ideology. An important part of the social indicator program of research must therefore be to provide a *framework* of analysis that is not, itself, value specific.[2] It is desperately easy to condition one's analysis in advance. A recent example comes from a paper by Allan Maslove (1975) who states three principal criteria for the design of indicators of which the first is: 'to develop indicators to guide government policy formation that, at the same time, are directly relevant to individual utility. In other words, indicators should be quantitative measures of attributes that directly affect human welfare; *they should be arguments in individual utility functions*' (Maslove, 1975, 8, italics added). Thus, in what seems to be a fairly innocuous economic interpretation of the proper function of social indicators, we have a criterion that commits us to a particular value-laden approach.

If the criterion means more than the commonplace observation that only individuals choose (*viz.* have utility functions), which we presume it does, it seems that since he fails to specify *which* individuals' utility functions are the

---

2 I shall not here enumerate what seem to me to be the bad parts of the 'radical' view. For those with sufficient interest, my views can doubtless be inferred from what is to come.

relevant ones we may infer that the ones in Maslove's mind are the consumers' utility functions conventionally taken as the point of departure in economic analysis. If we may not infer this, then it is not clear that any meaning at all can be attached to this 'criterion.' Thus, what may seem at first blush to be a fairly uncontroversial assertion not only commits us to a particular view about who should be the arbiters of social policy (insofar as it commits us to anything at all) but also, as a criterion, denies the legitimacy of enquiring about what must be a fundamental discussion in all social indicator programs: namely whose values are to count and how can a methodology be devised which does not prejudice the selection of any out of the great variety of answers that could be given to such a question?

One of the best ways of quelling the fears of the sceptics, whatever their party, is by not claiming too much. Modesty has the attractive property that it discourages premature counter-reaction against the social indicators program at the early practical hurdles. It is, of course, quite natural that enthusiasts should be enthusiastic and, indeed, they would be less than consistent were they otherwise. Oversell usually implies overclaim, however, and can frequently take subtle forms.

Henderson's otherwise excellent review is a case in point. Consider:

the need to develop social indicators ... is quite generally accepted as a result of a number of factors ... One of these has been the clear emergence during the past few years of certain social tensions and pressures ... These tensions and pressures have arisen, in part, from the rapid urbanization of our society, with increasing concentration of population in our largest urban centres; from the considerable shift over time in the industrial structure of the economy towards a larger service sector and towards the greater production of nonmarket goods and services, resulting in changing human resource requirements; from the desire of various minority ethnic groups to achieve a status in society equivalent to that of the major groups; from the unsettling effects of some aspects of technological change; and from changing social mores, brought about, in part, by the continually increasing ease of communication. (Henderson, 1974, 8).

The quotation instantly establishes its writer as a 'goody,' as a reasonably dispassionate assessor of the social scene and with only a little stretching – as an optimist. Aside from this, however, the quotation is an example of counter-productive propaganda in the social indicators cause, for it asserts, as fact and with breathtaking lack of qualification, a whole set of unknown causal patterns. In fact we do not know the answers to questions as to whether "tensions and pressures" have increased in the last twenty years. They seem to have changed, but even then in a way hard to describe, let alone quantify. It is not clear that the tensions of a more urbanized (say) society are more or less than those of a less urbanized one. In any event it is far from clear why the pressures of one should tend to produce a demand for social indicators more than the pressures of another.

On closer examination it is simply not true that considerations such as these have 'made clear the need for social indicators.' Why not be more modest – and more honest – and observe what really does seem to be fact: namely that governments today are trying to do a lot more about social problems than they did in the past (whatever their reasons) and that it seems quite a good idea to evolve a structure of thinking in which policy might be developed and evaluated both by government and the public, Cassandras and Pollyannas, conservatives and radicals. In fact, Henderson does go on to present essentially this argument. It does good arguments no service, however, to reinforce them with false ones.

Another failing of which enthusiasm can make us victims is to pretend that the impossible is, actually, quite possible. When it comes to specifying the goals 'society' has the temptations are overwhelming. Not surprisingly, the ground is littered with victims.

Henderson, for example, begins his discussion of the issues involved (Henderson, 1974, chap. 3) with an admirable statement describing the complexity of and conflicts between objectives that individuals and organizations in society seem to have. The stage seems set for an exposition of the more prominent features and paradoxes of contemporary social choice theory (Arrow, 1963; Sen, 1970). Instead, and despite his own caution, the subsequent paragraph launches into a set of assertions about basic human 'needs,' 'civilized needs' and quotes, apparently with approval, Maslow's five categories of need and their ranking (Maslow, 1954). Thus having asserted that conflicts exist over the desired ends in life, he proceeds to identify some unambiguous (if necessarily general) goals and even to assign them relative (and presumably unchanging) weights of importance.

The OECD approach to this problem is a shining beacon of clear-headed sense.[3]

Although there is no simple and easy way to clearly limit the concept of social well-being, it is even less easy to break it down into its component parts and specify these in such a way that they become tangible, measurable and manageable.

3 The OECD group, of course, has better reason than most to take seriously conflicts of interest, in view of the clientele which it serves.

The main problems appear to be the following: (a) The identification of components of well-being touches on basic questions about what is valuable in life. How can value-differences be reconciled beyond the level of generalities? (b) The concept implies (could imply, at least according to some interpretation) standard setting, i.e., below a certain standard there is no, or very little, well-being; above the standard there is sufficient or much well-being. The question then arises: 'Who decides such standards?' (c) Historical developments and cultural values may differ so much between nations, and even within nations, that attempts to make the concept operational universally may be meaningless.

In fact, the whole issue is fraught with value judgments and the values involved are of such a fundamental nature that differences might not be easily resolved.

To avoid value implications, an attempt has been made to specify social well-being by a strictly scientific method, which is presumed to have universal application. Efforts to identify 'basic human needs' have been made in this way. Unfortunately, no such attempts have so far resulted in anything very concrete, and it is doubtful that they ever will. There are good philosophical grounds for denying even the possibility that they might, except if one also admits 'basic human values,' and that poses the old value problem again. (OECD, 1976, 6-7)

The OECD approach was to try to identify the shared value judgments of member countries' ministerial representatives. Since this seems an attractive way out of the dilemmas noted, we should note its possible justifications and limitations. It may be justified either because the indicators are developed for policy makers and therefore the values for those responsible for policy are the relevant ones. Alternatively, it may be argued that these are true 'social' values by virtue of the fact that the members of society are willing to delegate decisions concerning them to persons called 'ministers' who are ultimately accountable to these same members of society. The former of these has appeal, particularly to those of a pragmatic bent, while the latter raises questions that are best deferred to a later point (chapter three).

In the end, the choice of decision-maker runs the risk of being an arbitrary one either imposed institutionally (as in the case of OECD) or according to some set of rules that one wishes to impose on oneself. The prejudices of the present author are that it is improper for the arbiter of values to be the analyst himself – there has been no theory of society since the divine rights of kings that embodied the perception of the welfare of a society in one man (and none, ever, that thought it should be embodied in a social scientist!). Perhaps the closest one can get to identifying the goals of 'society' is to identify goals that are literally shared by each and every member of society, if such goals exist. Less austerely restrictive[4] than this consensus requirement is to select those goals that seem to be regarded as important by major groups in society, even if they do not figure prominently in ministerial utterances. Potentially more radical (because less acceptable to most members of society) would be the selection of a set of goals held by some minority group notable for their sanctity, responsibility, toughness, socialism, or whatever. The problem here is choosing the criterion that should determine which of the many potential such groups will be selected.

For better or worse, the procedure adopted here in the context of health will be to identify these goals that seem to be important judging from the extent to which they are voiced in public, subjected to public discussion, often mentioned by politicians and the press, *etc.* As a matter of fact this approach appears essentially to be that proposed by Henderson at a later point where (notwithstanding his initial discussion of the *a priori* choice of goals) principal 'goal areas' are based on a set put forward by the Economic Council of Canada. Subsequently, however, he identifies the more 'critical' of these areas according to some guesses about their likely significance in the future.

Establishing weights, or trade-offs, between indicators is not, in point of fact, a step that necessarily must be resolved prior to the collection of data that are suitable for use as indicators. Moreover, in the social indicator literature it is also a step that has, in general, received rather arbitrary and ill-considered treatment. As we shall see, the discussion of trade-offs in the health *index* literature has been of much greater sophistication and is of substantially greater interest than the discussion in the social *indicator* field.

Health indicators

In introducing the chapter specifying some indicators in health (and other areas of concern), the ECC struck an appropriately (given what we have already said) modest note: 'The principal indicators proposed are not intended, and should not be considered, to represent all facets of well-being in these areas, but only certain particular aspects of and all these imperfectly ... At present it is best to regard these indicators basically as monitoring devices that gauge the state of, and changes in, certain matters of importance to society and provide some initial insights of significance for policy planning' (ECC, 1974, 62).

Three indicators in particular were proposed for health: life expectancy at birth, infant mortality, and prime age mortality. For future development at both

---

4 Even the rather conservative Pareto criterion often used by economists to evaluate changes in social welfare does not assume a consensus as regards goals.

federal and provincial level, data concerning morbidity and utilization were strongly recommended. Emphasis was placed upon *treated* morbidity (64) rather than prevalence, as measured by the number of cases treated for each participant in the medical care insurance plans, broken down by ICDA category, age, sex, socio-economic group, and region. Utilization referred only to participation in medical insurance plans.

Probably preferable, if less easy to obtain, would be information on the underlying morbidity of the population itself. It is well-known that a substantial part of the *treatable* sickness in the community is, in fact, never treated since the individuals in questions never make the initial necessary contact with a physician. This is the aptly named submerged part of the 'iceberg' of sickness in society, which is almost certainly of significantly greater importance in a society concerned with minimizing ill-health (out of given resources) than the hypochondriacal 'wastes' that are sometimes alleged and seem to be more prominent in public discussion of the effectiveness of medical care programs in the popular and medical press.

Indeed if social indicators are to fulfill the promise that some believe them to hold out it is important that their initial design should not be constrained by current or anticipated data availability. The indicators that are chosen may turn out to require an entirely new data base. Whether it is regarded as 'worth' creating such a new base should, of course, depend upon its cost relative to the value of the indicators. To tailor the design of indicators to a presumption that it would *not* be worth generating entirely new data seems, however, an illegitimately premature judgment, and one that denies the possibility of making the relevant one concerning the value of indicators designed as precisely as possible for their purposes.

This point of view has been well-articulated by the OECD:

since it is the deficiency in the information base available to governments that gave impetus to the search for valid social indicators, an OECD programme based primarily on existing data could not be expected to produce useful practical results. The OECD Social Indicator Programme is not constrained by any preconceived notions about data systems. The objective is first to specify the data requirements as explicitly as possible, and subsequently to try to fill them ... Notwithstanding the imperfections at each stage [of practical implementation], emphasis remains on the deductive approach (from programme level to data level) in the belief that it is more fruitful to first attempt to ask the right question than to suit the question to what may be the perfect answer. (OECD, 1976, 8-10)

Such an approach in Britain has led to a set of questions being incorporated into the general household survey concerning the recent health experiences of households which, for the first time, has created for that country a routine social survey statistical picture of morbidity that is independent of the institutions of the health care sector.

The concerns itemized in the OECD programme have, after considerable discussion and alteration, been settled as: (a) the probability of a healthy life through all stages of the life cycle, and (b) the impact of health impairments on individuals. These have been further subdivided, each into two sub-concerns as follows: (ai) length of life; (aii) healthfulness of life; (bi) quality of health care in reducing pain and restoring functional capabilities; (bii) extent of universal distribution in the delivery of health care.

The proposed indicators for these concerns, together with their justifications are as follows:
(ai) 1. Life expectancy at ages 1, 20, 40, 60; 2. perinatal mortality. (aii) 3. Proportion of predicted future of life to be spent in a state of disability on the part of those individuals not disabled as a result of a permanent impairment, at ages 1, 20, 40, 60; 4. Proportion of persons disabled as a result of a permanent impairment in selected age brackets. (bi) 5. Maternal mortality; 6. average delay between occurence of an emergency event and appropriate treatment; 7. average delay between awareness of functional disturbance of a non-emergency nature and appropriate treatment; 8. economic accessibility.

Life expectancy (1) was chosen rather than average age of death on the grounds that it is independent of external factors such as migration and age-structure of the population. Life expectancy at age one is a better indicator of longevity than life expectancy at birth. Moreover, special concern is customarily felt for the life-chances of the very young which warrants their being treated separately.

Perinatal mortality (still births and deaths in the first week of life as a proportion of all still and live births) (2) was chosen mainly on the grounds that most deaths in the first year of life occur in the first week.

Indicators 3 and 4 take us to the very heart of the problem of building social indicators of health. These two are, on an appropriate definition of 'disability,' the relevant concepts of morbidity in social policy. Because the issues raised are so large and so all pervasive, we shall postpone their discussion until chapter four.

The OECD program takes the admirable view that the quality of a programme can be assessed only by reference to its outcome (and not by reference to the quantity or quality of its inputs). The particular difficulty that this raises, however, for the early development of indicators is that health status is affected by many more things than the health services alone. To isolate their effect would require the development and empirical estimation of a model of ill health that attributed changes in status to changes in the many possible variables that affect it. Maternal mortality (5) was chosen on the basis that, although it is not independent of the housing, education, nutrition, etc., of pregnant women, it is nevertheless a statistic that may (with due caution) be supposed to vary more strongly with respect to medical services supplied than to other variables. A disadvantage of this statistic alone (aside from the absence of a proper model of causation of the mortality) is the relatively small number of deaths from this cause in developed countries: time trends and interregional comparisons have therefore to be interpreted with caution.

At the time of its writing the OECD report had not defined 'appropriate treatment.' As an interim method of quantifying (6) and (7), it proposed, moreover, to measure distance of residence from hospitals, GPs, and pharmacies rather than time delays between the location of the incident and treatment (which seems, in a mobile community whose members often work at substantial distances from their residences, a very poor proxy – though one for which *providers* may have much sympathy since its use would tend to locate their jobs in residential areas!) The measure proposed for economic accessibility (8) was: $D - C / D - E$, where D is disposable income net of household expenditure of health insurance; C is the (factor) cost of health services consumed; and E is household net expenditure on health services. The ratio is claimed to measure the proportionate reduction in income available for non-health service consumption if the full cost of services currently used had to be paid rather than the expenditures actually incurred. This assumes that C and E are independent – which in aggregate they cannot be, for *someone* must pay the premiums for health insurance, or the taxes that finance health care! The report in fact refers to the benchmark as being the prices obtaining in a free market though it is not at all clear what operational meaning is to be attached to this (other than current unit costs of production). The larger the reduction in financial burden on a household, the smaller the value taken by this indicator (assuming that $E \leqslant D$ and $E \leqslant C$, its maximum value is one and its minimum value is minus infinity). Unfortunately, its value also becomes smaller the higher the cost of providing the care: for example, for a course of medical care whose cost was equal to household income the indicator's value would be zero *regardless* of the expenditure actually laid out by the household. Such eventualities are, with many contemporary procedures, by no means unduly fanciful. The possibility of negative values in this indicator raises several problems of interpretation: for example, with $C > D$ the smaller is E the less negative the index.

It is worth also looking at the consequences of supposing $C = E$. Here the index takes a value of unity (as is to be expected in an index using the 'market' as benchmark) regardless of the size of D implying that in the 'free market' accessibility is equal independently of income – a view to which no one at OECD actually subscribes!

There are doubtless many ways in which these difficulties may become ironed out. For our purposes, the principal interest of the OECD program lies in the recognition of 'disability' as a relevant measure of health status, the importance of the time duration of the disability, and of measures of disability (including death as one of the more ultimate kinds of disability!) that are based upon the *communities being served* rather than the *institutions serving them* which is currently the typical statistical basis of most morbidity data. The latter emphasis avoids two particular difficulties that exist with most extant data sources: (*a*) increased patient throughput (which presumably implies that a higher proportion of 'needs' are being met) commonly suggests that 'need' has increased; (*b*) the data fail to pick up those needs that are not processed by institutions. Each of these features will, in subsequent chapters, be seen as of crucial importance to the satisfactory design of health indicators.

The OECD programme is also close in spirit to the federal government's *A New Perspective* (Lalonde, 1974), whose concept of the 'health field,' for example, 'identifies requirements for health without regard to the niceties of professional, or sectoral boundaries' (63) and which also advocated a regular national health survey (now termed the Canada Health Survey) of disease prevalence *and health status*. We shall, of course, have more to say both about *A New Perspective* and the Canada Health Survey in later chapters.

HEALTH INDEXES

Concern with what we have termed health 'indexes' to distinguish them (or, rather, their historical development) from health indicators has followed a quite different rationale and development and, for the most part, has involved a rather different set of people. We have already observed that the health index literature has tended to focus on the micro (or program-specific) dimensions of health measurement. What is more, whereas health indicator development has occurred in the context of the development of a general scheme for social indicators, the index developments have occurred most intensively (to say no more) in the health territory. So far as I am aware, there is no parallel development in other areas of public concern such as education or housing.

This has had two profound consequences: one in terms of methodology and the other in terms of the disciplinary background of those who have contributed most to index development.

Whereas the methodological inspiration for social indicators was typically derived from concern to monitor the 'state and condition' of society, recognizing the deficiencies of both the macroeconomic data and the corresponding models (developed mainly by economists), the methodology of indexes was derived from specific concerns about the efficient management of health care. Thus, while the social indicator movement has at times become ensnared in philosophical and ethical questions concerning the proper objectives of society, the index movement has mostly been able to avoid these, concerning itself instead with the apparently more tractable question of how the outcomes of medical interventions are measured. This is at once a strength and a weakness of this literature. A strength in that much progress and experimentation has actually taken place into various forms of measurement; a weakness in that the avoidance of some of the difficult conceptual issues in indicators is really illusory: they have been ignored, on the whole, rather than avoided.

Related to this has been the disciplinary distinction between the two. Whereas social indicators have principally been developed by social scientists in economics, political science, and sociology, index development owes most to the work of medical, operations research, and biostatistical scientists. This again has reinforced the methodological differences in the history of the two types of measure, with the social scientists being highly preoccupied with abstract discussion of 'social welfare functions,' aggregation problems and models of society, while index researchers have focused more on engineering-type relationships which lend themselves more directly to empirical application. Increasingly, however, the index literature has confronted more explicitly the issues that have preoccupied the indicator literature though there is unfortunately, it seems, relatively little evidence of the two streams of research coming together to learn from one another.

Although the bulk of work on indexes has been done by non-economists, its principal context has been provided nevertheless by cost-benefit or cost-effectiveness analysis of alternative ways of doing things. In using these terms we have in mind their conventional meanings. Cost-benefit analysis refers to a procedure by which all the costs and benefits of alternative programs (not necessarily mutually exclusive programs) are compared so that those which are, in a special sense, most 'profitable' for society may be identified. Cost-effectiveness refers to the comparison of alternative ways of doing essentially the 'same' things so that those which are, again in a special sense, least costly for society may be identified.

The special and distinctive features of the economic approach in these techniques lies in its treatment of futurity via a discounting procedure (with which we shall not be concerned here) and in the concepts of cost and benefit which are employed. The notion of cost is *opportunity cost*, the foregone benefit of using a resource (whether human or non-human) in the way proposed rather than *either* in its most valued alternative use (which is the relevant notion for a fully general efficiency study) *or* in its expected alternative use, i.e., the employment it would be expected to have if the proposal is not adopted (which is the notion most commonly adopted in practical studies) and which involves the analyst neither in the (impossible) task of identifying the truly most valued alternative use out of all those that are potentially possible nor in the act of faith which supposes that, say, the current use (or any other) actually *is* the most valuable. Such an approach involves us immediately in scepticism concerning cash expenditures and market prices, for there is no general reason to suppose that these measure accurately the opportunity cost to society. For example, if a planned project utilizes resources of which there is believed to be a shortage (in the sense that at the going wage more are demanded than are available) then the current wage actually paid represents an *understatement* of the cost of transferring resources from their existing use to the proposed one. If the plan will use manpower that would be expected otherwise to be unemployed, although a positive wage will have to be paid, these resources will in fact be withdrawn from no alternative productive use, so from the point of view of the rest of society there is a *zero* opportunity cost. If the plan will incolve costs that do not fall on the budget of the agency funding expenditures (for example, a program of early discharge from hospital that raises household costs) likewise these are generally reckoned as relevant social opportunity costs. Implicit in the foregoing are value judgments relating to *whose* valuation of the alternatives foregone is to be given weight. The typical value judgment employed is to assert that, at the least, the values should include those external to the agency in question and, except when a plausible case why not can be put, should include *all* potential alternative values in society (for example, the value of foregone output of children above statutory school leaving age would be included but *not* of children below that age-level even though they could be usefully employed.[5]

On the benefit side, in principle *all* benefits, to whomsoever they accrue (unless, again, plausible exceptions can be urged — such as, perhaps, those who are deemed to be unable to form a coherent view for themselves about benefit) are reckoned. It is, of course, on the benefit side that the health index literature

5 Such an exclusion would not, of course, be made in a cost-benefit study of the merits of raising or lowering the statutory school-leaving age.

has focused, for an adequate measure of health outcomes — and their valuation — has been the principal lacuna in empirical studies both of the cost-effectiveness type (which require a *unit* to be costed) and of the cost-benefit type (which require units not only to be costed but also valued).

Since the index literature has an extremely rich set of possible measures of health status, of much greater subtlety and complexity than the social indicators literature, we shall not embark on a synoptic account of it in the present chapter. Instead, we shall devote the whole of chapters five and six to a review of social indicators, with a view in particular to identifying the kind of value-concentrating increasingly on Ontario as we go along. In chapters four and five we shall explore critically the conceptual foundations both of these indexes and of social indicators, with a view in particular to identifying the kind of value judgments that must, of necessity be made, and also the necessary logical steps that are common to both.

In subsequent chapters we shall also drop the distinction made here between 'indexes' and 'indicators' in favour of the more general term 'health status measures.' One reason for this is that the micro-macro distinction in their use has never in fact been faithfully followed — nor is there any reason, of course, why this heuristic device should have been followed. In particular, the public health literature has commonly discussed 'indices' and 'indexes' at a highly aggregate level (e.g., Stouman and Falk, 1936). A second, much more important, reason is that the use of a single term emphasizes the common conceptual issues which underly both macro and micro measures and which will be a major concern in subsequent chapters.

3
The public interest
and private interests

The enjoyment of the highest attainable standard of health is one of the fundamental rights of every human being without distinction of race, religion, political belief, economic or social condition. *Constitution of the World Health Organization*

The public interest in health has been typically manifested by community action to deal with health problems that the individual was incapable of managing himself. In recent decades, a number of factors have enlarged the scope of the public interest and given it new force and cogency. The first is a deepening of our humanitarian concern for our fellows ... We seem [also] ... to ... believe that an individual family should not have to bear alone the full cost of risks that could happen to anyone of us ... There is yet ... the appalling social and economic cost to Canada of ill-health, proving that the family and the nation pay heavily in terms of lost production for failure to make available to all Canadian citizens the standard of health service we know how to provide. *Royal Commission on the Health Services*

The basic objective of Ontario's health services plan is to provide and maintain for residents of the province a state of physical, mental and social well-being, including the prevention or treatment of disease or infirmity, to the extent possible given the resources that are available. *Report of the Health Planning Task Force, Ontario*

The distinction between the public interest and the private interest is one that is commonly met in discussions of the proper role of government and the extent to which it should monitor and control the resource use patterns of society including the extent to which the government should own resources. Since the distinction between the two kinds of interest is fundamental to the argument of this book and since there are many possible distinctions that can be (and are) made, this chapter makes clear the sense in which the distinction will be used here, and indicates some of the broader consequences of the distinction which will be taken up in greater detail in subsequent chapters. The present chapter begins at the most general level and progressively narrows down the issues as they arise in the context of health care. In this way it is hoped that the underlying approach adopted here will be made as fully explicit as possible.

The fundamental point of departure is the assertion that the individual citizen is the origin of *both* the notion of a private *and* a public interest. We shall not find it necessary to admit that the public interest is a perception of social desiderata by any set of individuals possessing special moral, intellectual, religious, class, or genealogical characteristics, though frequently decisions concerning the public interest will be delegated to a relatively few persons, whose special characteristics may include the fact that they have been elected by other individuals for this purpose and are ultimately accountable to them for their decisions, or have been appointed by those who have been elected.

An individual's private interest, interpreted in the most austerely restrictive sense, is an interest which is his and his alone, a purpose pursued by the individual which is neither shared nor opposed by any other individual. Note that even in this most restricted sense, however, the purely private interests of individuals may conflict indirectly, insofar as the pursuit of individual purposes may use up resources that other individuals are deprived of as they pursue their own private ends. The classic way of resolving this conflict over resource use (but not over purposes) is, in western societies, via the use of markets. A famous theorem of economics shows, indeed, that if all interests are private in the sense used here, then a competitive market will ensure that (given some initial distribution of purchasing power) resources will become so distributed that each is used for those private purposes that are most highly valued by individuals. In the language of utilitarianism: the sum total of utility in society will be maximized. In the language of modern economics: a Pareto optimum will obtain.

It is not intended to place any substantial faith in this theorem for the purposes of the present study, however, for the transparent reason that the circumstances for which the theorem is asserted to be (logically) true apply neither in general nor, for our own purposes, in the health territory. It is, however, immediately apparent that no society could exist of the sort described that was composed *solely* of private interests, for if the normative judgment is made that 'its' well-being is to be made as high as possible, then so long as the 'society' in question consists of more than one individual out of the total number of individuals who could be considered eligible, even the society of atomistic individuals pursuing strictly private ends has public or collective interests. Notably they concern the specification, allocation, policing, and enforcement of the private property rights which are the *sine qua non* of the market system, and which are the 'things' that are traded in such a system as conflict over who shall use which resources becomes resolved in the market place.

Not much reflection is required, moreover, before it is apparent that such purely private interests rarely exist. The society described above requires but one busybody, or one do-gooder, prude, friend, enemy and, so long as that person counts as a member of society, then the whole fabric crumbles; for the interests of any individual now become the interests, in some degree, or counter to the interests, in some degree, of the busybody, etc.[1]

Moreover, there are two other major individual sources of public interest. The first is that individuals clearly have an interest in some of the collective attributes of their society: for example, individuals are manifestly not indifferent to the income levels, absolute or relative, of other members of society, so there is an individualistic foundation for public concern about income distribution and redistribution. Income redistribution has therefore the characteristics of 'publicness' in the technical sense that a given level of inequality (or equality) in incomes confronts every member of the community.

The second source arises out of technological interdependencies between individual units: the classic case of the smoky factory chimney dumping soot and smells on neighbourhoods. Given private property rights and zero transaction costs, the Coase theorem (Coase, 1960) predicts with impeccable logic that the decentralized market mechanism will produce an efficient outcome. Where, however, transaction costs are positive and large numbers of individuals are affected by the 'spillover' once again individuals may find it in the private interest to delegate collective decision-making to some selected representatives. Once again a *public* interest arises.

Clearly, the preferred (by the individuals in a society) balance between public (i.e., collective) and private decision-making will be determined within the framework outlined here, by a variety of technical characteristics concerning the extent of interdependencies of the sort described, the importance ascribed to them, the relative advantages (costs) of collective and private decision

1 Such a general approach, while now quite fashionable among economist studying problems of philanthropy and externalities was formulated quite a long time ago by Allen (1932).

procedures, and ethical – sometimes constitutional – views about the 'legiti-macy' of the interdependency in question. Provided that democracy is not too 'imperfect' such a balance will presumably be reflected in the actual arrange-ments adopted by society.

'Legitimacy' raises questions that involve quintessential political value-judgments about which the economist has no special right to express a preference. Society seems to take a consensus view in some specific cases: the kind of music one listens to privately is judged an entirely private matter; the state of one's health, even though it may involve no communicable disease, is regarded as a public as well as a private concern. There is, however, some ambiguity about other aspects: behaviour that is purely private in all respects save that it may affect one's health and hence provide the basis for collective control of, e.g., one's smoking habits or whether or not one wears a seat-belt in automobiles. The resolution of such questions determines people's constitutional rights – more specifically, individual property rights and the extent and manner in which they may be exchanged.

From these general considerations we may turn to the appropriate interpreta-tion of the public interest in individuals' health status. In order to avoid the potential controversy inherent in including every aspect of the division – and possible conflict – between the public and the private interest, we focus only on those areas that are most relevant for the subsequent discussion of health status measurement and health care planning.

The relevant sources of public interest in health care that have been chiefly noted in the literature, and/or can be inferred from it and from public statements of governments, may be summarized under the following heads: (i) communicable disease, (ii) financial burden, (iii) geographical distribution, (iv) health status.

COMMUNICABLE DISEASE

This is the 'classic' case of the public interest in health care and has been extensively analysed in the economic literature (e.g., Klarman, 1965; Weisbrod, 1961) and it provides either the explanation of, or the justification for, (depending on the nature of the analysis) government programs of public health, inoculation, vaccination, and some other preventive and screening programs.

The essence of the argument runs as follows: in decisions concerning an individual's health he will take such precautions and remedial actions that he considers best, bearing in mind the costs and the benefits to himself. If the price of, say, immunization is the same to all individuals but the benefits they perceive vary, then only those individuals for whom the subjective benefits exceed the cost will immunize. Arranging individuals in descending order by benefit, the argument may be depicted in Figure 1.

We suppose that the private value placed by individuals upon an immunization is distributed normally about a mean[2], so that placing individuals in descending order of valuation, a curve similar in shape to *BEb* in Figure 1 may be drawn. Beyond *Og*, the remaining individuals place a *negative* value upon the program (e.g., for religious reasons, because of strong risk aversion[3], or simply because of subjective costs associated with injections, doctors' visits, etc.) Given a cost (equals price to the patient) represented by *aE* only those individuals whose valuation exceeds this sum will voluntarily present themselves, viz. *Oa* per cent. In the absence of any public interest elements, and provided a number of other conditions are met, *Oa* may be regarded as the optimal degree of coverage for a preventive program, where to increase coverage further would cause social costs to exceed social benefits at the margin.

With immunization, however, spillover benefits do occur: the higher the proportion of persons vaccinated the smaller the probability that the remainder will contract the disease. This benefit is not captured in the curve *BEb* nor in the marginal cost curve *Cc* (assumed fully to include social costs). We suppose that these external (marginal) benefits accruing to the remainder of the community follow the shape of the dotted curve Ob^e which becomes zero when $(n - 1)/n$ per cent of the population of n persons are immunized. When added to the internal benefits upon which we suppose individuals to base their private calculations, the community benefit curve BE^1b^1b is obtained.[4] This curve intersects the *Cc* line to the right of the 'private' equilibrium, indicating that the 'social' optimum, determined by equality between the benefits received by the marginal individual *plus* the additional benefits accruing to all non-vaccinated persons and the cost of vaccinating a marginal individual, implies a higher rate of immunization of the community: *Of* per cent rather than *Oa* per cent.

In the figure as shown it is to be noted that the optimal coverage (*Of*) falls short of that which would be voluntarily taken at zero price (*Og*). In fact, a marginal price of *fh* per patient would be required to ensure the optimal rate of coverage by voluntary means. By the same token, 100 per cent coverage would require a marginal subsidy of *OS*.

---

2 This assumption seems plausible but is not necessary.

3 There is a risk with some vaccinations of actually contracting the disease in question and fatalities are known occasionally to occur. It may be that no finite price would compensate some individuals in the tail of the distribution.

4 We do not assume that expected utility is independent of the number of others to be immunized.

Figure 1

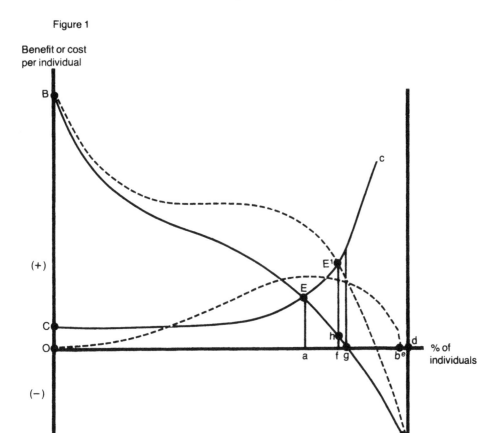

In practice, of course, only points such as *E* and *g* are actually observable in the real word (depending on the price set) while the benefits represented by the curves drawn in broken lines are not empirically observable – at least not very readily so. Governmental authorities in consultation with epidemiological and other experts form a judgment about the degree to which there is 'not enough' coverage and evaluate whether an extension would be 'worthwhile.' In practice this usually amounts to a decision to make the service free of charge to all patients and to finance it out of general revenues. In Figure 1, such a policy (assuming zero income effects) results in a small over-provision (by *fg*) though it could also, of course, result in under-coverage. Given, however, the costs of acquiring sufficient information to identify the true optimum, and of operating a subsidy system (or of coercing individuals) to ensure that it is attained, such a policy may be viewed as a reasonable second best.

We have dwelt on this reasoning at some length since the arguments adduced in this case bear a close resemblance to all the standard arguments adduced for public intervention in the health territory, as we shall see. Also as we shall see, certain implications for health planning and, in particular, information needs, are implied by them.

At this stage it is instructive to identify the principal value judgments that are inherent in the approach. At a later stage in the book we shall see that these value judgments are of central importance for the definition and design of a proper information system. Those judgments which we seek to identify now are as follows:

(1) It is assumed (as is conventional in welfare economics) that the benefits ascribed by individuals to the services they receive are the relevant benefits in deciding how much of a service should be provided and under what terms.

(2) It is further assumed that there is some not negligible set of individuals (set 1) to whom value judgment (1) applies.

(3) There may also be other individuals whose use of a service, or whose state of health, yields benefits either of a direct physical kind (as with reduced incidence of disease) or more abstractly (e.g., because of humanitarian feelings) to those individuals in set 1 defined by value judgment (2). This new set of individuals (set 2) will normally overlap with set 1 but may also include individuals excluded from set 1. For example, children's appreciation/valuation of benefits is often regarded as irrelevant in health care (and in many other areas too), so they are excluded from set 1. They normally, however, figure prominently in set 2, since their state of health (etc.) is of great concern to parents (etc.) who are normally members of set 1. The benefits to persons in set 2, as evaluated by those in set 1, are to be found in both curves $BE'b'$ and the dotted curve connecting O and b^e.

(4) The approach takes a somewhat cavalier attitude to the distribution of the costs and benefits of the program. Suppose the immunization program is financed out of general taxation. It thus follows that the value of the service to some may be less than the tax share in its financing attributed to them. The analysis assumes that the uncompensated 'losses' of such persons may be set against the gains to others on a dollar-for-dollar basis. In any case, the benefit curve of Figure 1 is based upon 'willingness-to-pay' and is hence conditioned by the existing income and wealth distributions which may or may not be regarded as sacrosanct. A more sophisticated approach would introduce more complicated value judgments concerning variable weights to be attached to gains and losses. But where the legitimate source of such weights may be is a moot point. Having

no special competence in such a decision, the economist can offer only the dollar-for-dollar assumption (viz. unitary weights) as provisional, to be suitably modified where appropriate with those having legitimate authority to do so.

(4′) As an alternative to (4) one could treat the distributional issues as something entirely separate from the 'efficiency' issues based upon the 'willingness-to-pay' principles underlying the analysis. This has much to commend it. Distributional issues tend to confuse the efficiency analysis, even to render people doubtful about its acceptability (as far as it goes). Moreover, the use of distributional weights in efficiency analysis tends to oversimplify the genuine concerns in distribution. This alternative approach gives both elements in the public decision a clear role. Decisions will be based upon a judicious balancing of the two, with neither 'efficiency' nor 'justice' alone dominating the other.

FINANCIAL BURDEN

There can be little doubt that the principal driving force behind the postwar changes that most advanced countries have made in their health care financing methods has had its source in the feeling (by set 1 individuals) that individuals (in either set 1 or set 2) should not be denied the opportunity, for reasons of financial hardship, of maintaining a reasonable health status.

We may decompose this issue into its two obvious parts: concern about financial burden and concern about health status. Public discussion as well as public policy has concentrated overwhelmingly on the first of these. The second, however, is of no less importance and its implications are, as we shall see, of profound consequence. We shall take each in turn.

The vexed issues involved in answering questions concerning the proper role (if any at all) of the patient in financing health care services in Ontario have been dealt with at length elsewhere and it is the purpose here neither to review them comprehensively nor to survey in any detail the few pieces of extant relevant evidence bearing on some of them. Traditionally, the argument has centred upon the demand side: the deterrent effect of user-charges, copayments, deductibles, etc., and their 'justice' or 'fairness' in terms of both of the distribution of the burden of financing the system and of the distribution of delivered health care services. In particular, concern over the rising cost, both absolute and relative, of medical care has led to a reawakening of interest in user-charges, partly for deterrent purposes, partly to raise funds additional to those raised through premiums and general taxation, and partly for purposes of educating the public about the cost of care.

After a brief discussion again of some of these issues, we suggest an alternative approach which places a new kind of emphasis on the supply side and which offers, *prima facie,* an alternative avenue of control that conflicts less with the objective of health care policy.

One of the great difficulties confronting analysts and policy makers in this highly emotional area of debate is that it is not at all easy to see how the issues can be separated out neatly into boxes labelled respectively 'efficiency' and 'equity'. Thus, while the two quotations cited at the beginning of this chapter may seem rather unambiguously to relate, for the most part, to notions of equity or social justice, many economists would feel strongly inclined to describe the concerns there described as 'spillovers' and proceed to describe allocations of resources that were 'efficient' but which embodied in them the humanitarian (etc.) concerns which are undoubtedly at the heart of health service politics.

The first thing, then, which we have to emphasize is that health care which is provided free at the point of use is not necessarily by virtue of this fact alone, inefficiently provided. Indeed, if it is the case that the Canadian people in general, and Ontarians in particular, do feel a humanitarian concern for one another and do feel that a unique distinguishing mark of Canadian citizenship is contained in the sentiment that all have equal access to equally good care, then absence of patient charges becomes the likely characteristic of an efficient system.

A corollary of this is, however, often overlooked: the personal distribution of *health care* should be completely independent of the personal distribution of *income* and the personal distribution of *contributions.* While these latter may be perfectly legitimate questions of public interest, the nature of that interest is quite independent of, and should be discussed independently of, questions concerning the distribution of health care. This is not to argue that distributional questions should be ignored. On the contrary, they should receive more explicit attention than is customary.

Policy concerns about distributional questions may be divided into concerns about generalized economic power (income or wealth distributions) and more specific distributions (such as that of health status). *Part* of the concern with the former may be attributable to the fact that there are many sets of the latter (health, education, housing, nutrition, etc.) To this extent they interact. But just as achieving a satisfactory (whatever that may be) distribution of economic power may leave residual dissatisfaction with some in-kind distributions so a satisfactory set of in-kind distributions may leave residual dissatisfaction with the distribution of economic power. Both types are important, but health policy, while having implications for general redistribution policy, should focus primarily upon the distribution of health status.

As a general rule, both economists and social reformers (who are not always the same people!) focus their interest on income distributions, to the near exclusion of all other kinds of distribution. While income distributions (and redistributions) are, of course, of great importance they are an extremely poor description of the totality of man's concern about the distribution of goods and services[5] in society. Indeed, were they the only concern, then public policy need concern itself only with making cash transfers among citizens. But public policy of course does not do that, taking instead a profound interest in the in-kind distribution of education, housing, health, and so on *as well as* in-cash distributions.[6]

If, then, the principles which should govern the distributions of health care are different from those which should govern the personal distribution of income, it follows that attempts to recoup the costs of medical care from patients are likely to satisfy the principles of one only by offending against the principles of the other. Indeed, since it is known that the elasticity of demand for care is not zero (that is why, of course, deterrent charges are sometimes proposed) and since it seems also to be a corollary of the nature of the public interest in health care distribution that its allocation should be entirely independent of the income of its recipients, it follows that user charges that deter (viz., marginal charges) will serve the health care objectives only by chance and may (depending on whether their burden falls regressively or not) also conflict with the usual principles of distribution in general. Thus, even a system of financing which was carefully designed to ensure so far as possible that utilization responded to charges only and *not* to the income of individuals, will likely conflict with the postulated distributional objectives – not the *income* distribution objective but the 'in-kind' health status distribution, for if the ideal is to make utilization follow the potential for improving health status (a notion to be much expanded later) there is no general presumption that charges of any kind will help towards this aim. Indeed, by discouraging utilization, they will likely detract from it: more sickness will simply remain undiagnosed.

---

5 Though they may, in conjunction with the wealth distribution, be a useful indicator of the distribution of economic power.

6 Economists' prejudices in this regard may partly stem from a well-established (but erroneous) theorem allegedly demonstrating the superiority of cash over in-kind transfers. Since this welfare theorem has as its corollary certain implications in positive economics, the problem remains, for those who accept it, of explaining why all countries seem to persist in adhering to a great variety of 'demonstrably inefficient' policies. The usual explanation is in terms of the irrationality of government or the imperfection of democracy: *ad hoc* devices whose use is customarily (and rightly) deplored in the explanation of market phenomena.

TABLE 1

Still-births and infant deaths to mothers in England and Wales aged under 25, (1959-63)

	Previous number of live and still-births		
	0	1 or 2	3 or More
Still-births per 1000 births			
Social classes I and II	10.5	8.6	5.1
Social class III	14.6	9.8	11.4
Social classes IV and V	15.6	10.4	13.2
Neo-natal deaths per 1000 live births			
Social classes I and II	9.6	8.8	12.8
Social class III	12.2	11.1	16.5
Social classes IV and V	13.3	12.1	16.3
Post neo-natal deaths per 1000 live births			
Social classes I and II	3.9	4.3	10.3
Social class III	4.4	9.2	17.3
Social classes IV and V	6.1	10.2	15.4

SOURCE: *Social Trends* 6, 1975, 26 (HMSO)
NOTE: The social class definitions used here are the broad occupational classifications used in the census. They are: I professional and similar occupations, II intermediate occupations, III skilled occupations (non-manual and manual), IV partly skilled occupations, V unskilled occupations.

At this stage we may emphasize two further important points. First, although the evidence on the 'deterrent effect' of price is patchy it is reasonably clear and bears out what one would expect (Beck, 1973, 1974). But this is not the end of the story. Price is but one of the factors affecting the demand for health services.[7] Depending on the precise content of the public interest in individuals' health, one may have to go a good deal further. In Britain, a country well-known for the absence of user-charges of any significance for the principal health services, there is evidence of variation in health status and health services utilization that would doubtless be of concern were they to be found in Canada (see Tables 1 and 2). Moreover, there is ample evidence from morbidity surveys that there is a high prevalence of disease in the community that is untreated (though treatable) and even unrecognized by the diseased person (Office of Health Economics, 1964). And this for a country showing similar values to those

7 The most comprehensive demand study to date is probably Grossman (1972).

TABLE 2

Use of health services by children up to age 7 (Great Britain, 1965)

Social class (of father)	(a) Visited a dentist	(b) been immunized against:		
		smallpox	polio	diphtheria
I	16	6	1	1
II	20	14	3	3
III (non-manual)	19	16	3	3
III (manual)	24	25	4	6
IV	27	29	6	8
V	31	33	10	11
All classes	23	23	5	6

Percentage of children who had never:

SOURCE: *Social Trends* 6, 1975, 27 (HMSO)

of Canadians and with a health care system of broadly comparable effectiveness (at least as measured by the crude indicators upon which we have to rely for such comparisons. In 1972, for example, the infant mortality rate in the UK was 17.6 against Canada's 17.1 and male and female life expectancies were 69.0 and 75.3 respectively in England and Wales against 68.8 and 75.2 in Canada).

The second point to emphasize is that the value judgments embodied in the general views described above are not necessarily those of the author[8] but are, instead, what he hopes are those to be inferred by reasonably detached inference from the public utterances of persons whose values are taken as broadly representative of Canadian public opinion as, for example, illustrated by the quotations at the beginning of this chapter.

Once again, however, we shall have to go a good way further than these, for, as is so often the way with broad declarations of good intent, the more closely one wishes to apply them to reality, the more elusive their operational meaning becomes.

To recapitulate the conclusions of the argument in this section, we find that, while concern about both the distribution of the costs of the health care system and the distribution of the services of that system are both manifestly areas of

8 Whose principal value judgment as a social scientist concerns the impropriety of social scientists inflicting their own value judgments on the rest of society: in short a value judgment about scientific method, not about social policy.

the public interest, the public interest in the two is not the same. We do not have to enquire too closely at this stage into the meaning of an intent such as 'to provide such services ... as ... will ensure that the best possible care is available to all Canadians,'[9] to infer that it does not include a requirement either that the poor sick should necessarily receive more care than the rich sick nor that the rich sick should necessarily contribute more to health care finance than the poor in general, the poor sick, or, indeed, the rich in general. What it manifestly does include, however, is the requirement that health service distribution should be related to whether individuals are (a) sick (or likely to become sick), and (b) Canadian.

In the economists' jargon of the preceding discussion of 'spillovers' in the immunization case, we are driven irresistibly to the conclusion that the health status of each and every individual has spillover effects upon the rest of us, a phenomenon that is legitimately regarded as justifying collective action to procure that distribution of health status which is preferred. This social interest lies in the provision of health services that have identifiable impact upon health status and that provide care for dependent persons. There is, on this argument, no general case for the public subsidy of ineffective care. Moreover, at the margin, society's collective decision-makers may decide that the social pay-off per dollar to (say) subsidized orthodontia – basically cosmetic procedures or, indeed, any procedures judged trivial in terms of their impact on health status – is lower than that to spending in other areas. It becomes, under such circumstances, the privilege of the rich to pay, if they so wish, for ineffective and trivial procedures: ineffective from a technical point of view; trivial from the collective, not necessarily from the individual, point of view.

As soon as it is seen that probably the most effective way of advancing this social interest is by running a health service that is, to all intents and purposes, free of charge, concern with the health status of others becomes even stronger; for the mechanism of the market, which is used to regulate the demands made by individuals upon the system as they seek to promote their healthfulness, is destroyed. Now society itself, and those decision-makers who act for it, need some indicators of what changes in healthfulness are being effected and, since not all possible beneficial changes can be effected out of given resources, a rationing criterion is needed.

A fundamental article of faith in the health status measurement literature is that the criterion must relate to health. A rational health sector needs health status indexes.

9 From the terms of reference of the Royal Commission on Health Services.

GEOGRAPHICAL DISTRIBUTION OF HEALTH RESOURCES

An important element in this concern for the health status of others – at least in Canada – has related to the geographical distribution of health care. In the words of the Hall Commission (Royal Commission on Health Services, 1964, 9): 'we cannot ignore the unequal distribution of resources, particularly of personnel, to meet our health needs ... if there ever was a time when Canadians in one section of our country could be oblivious to lower health standards elsewhere in Canada, that time is *not now*. There is clearly an overriding *national* interest in the health of Canadians wherever they reside ... It is necessary, therefore, to review the distribution of health resources – personnel and facilities – as a primary concern of the public interest.'

Unlike Britain, however, where a similar concern is also shown and where (but only recently) an explicit budget formula for equalizing per capita expenditures or real resources in the regions has been devised, the Commission recommended no explicit measures of this sort. There is, above all, one particular reason why such may have been the case.

The passage from the Commission's report that has just been quoted refers to the 'distribution of resources ... *to meet our health needs*' (my italics) and the addition of the italicized clause qualifies the relatively simple equality of *access* objective by clearly suggesting that, whatever 'needs' may precisely be, they are important in determining what the geographic pattern of resource distribution ought to be. It is all too easy to assert, but subsequently to forget at the planning level, that 'The purpose of health services is to preserve or improve the health of the people or minimize the consequences of ill health' (ibid., 139). As the Mustard report on health planning in Ontario said, 'where the need for services is greatest, few measures have been undertaken to influence the social and environmental causes of ill health and none in coordination with the provision of remedial services. In short, no plan has been developed for the delivery of health services in relation to the over-all needs of the population' (Task Force, 1974, 8). With regard to physicians, the report went on (66) to recommend the establishment of physician quotas for each district in the province – though the guidelines for determining these quotas were (judiciously perhaps) left unspecified.

It is clear that underlying these concerns for geographical equity in the distribution of health care resources is a still more profound concern which relates to the measurement of the health needs of the population, for there would manifestly remain grave injustices as well as inefficiency in a system that allocated its resources according to, say, the distribution of the population when the underlying morbidity characteristics of the population varied widely.

Indeed, as we shall argue in the next chapter, geographical equity *per se* makes little sense. What does make sense is the meeting of 'need' (provided, of course, that 'need' receives a suitable and operational definition). It is only to the extent that 'need' has a geographical dimension that geography gets into the picture at all. Just why this is so we shall explore at greater length in the subsequent two chapters.

DIRECT HEALTH STATUS

Public interest in the health status of individuals is, as we have tried to argue, the most important single reason for collective action in the organization and delivery of health services. At the same time, empirical knowledge of the health status of populations and individuals, of the impact on that status of medical (and other kinds of) intervention is remarkably thin and is often based upon acts of faith as one infers impacts, trends, etc., from cruder surrogates such as mortality data, or even from input information.

The importance of health status is manifest at many levels of policy concern. At one level we have the kind of comparison made by Cochrane whereby, for example, it appears that 'Canada gets a similar output [from its health services] to that of the United Kingdom with about double the input as regards money per head per annum' (Cochrane 1975, 281). At the opposite extreme from this highly aggregated kind of comparison we have the micro problems of clinical practice and medical research. In the words of one of Britain's most distinguished neurosurgeons:

Perhaps the most serious of all mis-directions of effort is the vigorous and sometimes prolonged treatment of patients with brain damage so extensive that, although death may be deferred, the postponement brings to the family and so society only misery and expense. This is *unsuccessful* treatment. While some patients recover to varying degrees, others are left as a human shell, awake but vacant, speechless and spastic and with no evidence of a functioning mind either receiving or projecting information ... [T]he wooly terms used by neurosurgeons to describe recovery ('worthwhile,' 'useful,' 'practical') ... [are] ... a serious hindrance when it comes to comparing the efficacy of different regimes of management and to stabilizing prognostic criteria. (Jennett, 1974)

In between these two extremes comes health status measurement as a tool to aid resource distribution. This has efficiency dimensions: presumably it is an objective of the health service to meet 'needs' efficiently. It also has equity dimensions: presumably greater 'needs' receive priority over lesser.

The traditional economic literature in health, especially at the theoretical level, is to be noted both for the assiduity with which it avoids emotive words like 'need' and also for the high level of abstraction at which it deals with the spillovers that are widely hypothesized to exist in health (both of the direct physical kind discussed earlier in the present chapter and, more generally, of the humanitarian kind that seem to be implied by the quotations at the beginning of this chapter).

It seems, however, not at all fanciful to suppose that the principal component of this spillover (whichever kind it may be) is in fact the health status of third parties: just as it is the health status of a potential disease carrier that causes the direct spillover, so it is the health status of other persons that is the object of humanitarian concern.

We should, however, point out that (plausible though it seems to be) this interpretation of the object of concern is not one that is frequently encountered in the economic literature. Here, the typical representation is of concern with health care consumption rather than health status. Thus, Pauly (1971, 21) argues: 'If an individual's consumption of medical care does provide benefit to others, this must mean, [sic] that at some level of consumption by that individual, other persons would be willing to pay for him to consume an additional unit of medical care'. In a similar view, Culyer (1971, 65)[10] argues that 'dropping the assumption of selfishness in human behaviour ... assume that of two classes of individual, rich and poor, the relatively low consumption of health services by the poor in the open market imposes external disutilities on the rich.' Lindsay (1969, 76) side-steps the issue as follows: 'What is desired among individuals demonstrating the same "medical need" is *more equal* treatment.'

The emphasis on care given rather than health status attained or altered through intervention is not unique to the economic literature. It is, nevertheless, an odd emphasis (especially for economists). For one thing it identifies the *output* of health services with their inputs (a practice that is not conducive to clear thinking about a sensible and fair allocation of resources). For another, it supposes that the public interest is as well met by an equal distribution of *ineffective* health care as it is by an equal distribution of *effective* health care,

10 Page references to this and Lindsay's article, quoted below, are to the reprinted versions in Cooper and Culyer (1973).

which appears an extremely implausible interpretation of the public interest as it has been expressed.

We therefore focus here directly upon the health status of individuals. A further advantage of this approach, as we shall see, is that it leads us directly into a consideration of the effectiveness of medical procedures and hence offers a further angle of attack upon the problem of containing health care expenditures. What we hope to have shown in this chapter is that the whole of the health status measurement movement can be interpreted not as an intellectually *arbitrary* approach to solving some of the pressing problems of the day, but rather as a logical outcome of quite conventional and traditional concepts of efficiency and fairness: hingeing crucially, it is true, upon the abstract concept of the "spillover" but offering the promise of putting some substantive and quantitative content into what can otherwise be only abstract and qualitative.

CONCLUSIONS

The interpretation of the public interest adopted here is one that is based upon a presumption that individuals are not indifferent to one another's states of health both because they may be physically affected and because of humanitarian concerns relating principally to the burden of the costs of medical care and directly to health status itself (viz. they care about others' health). We assume that these interests are institutionalized in a government which is accountable for its actions to the people, and even though we recognize that the perfect representation of these interests is not possible, yet we take the public utterances of governments and public bodies (some of which are quoted at the beginning of this chapter) as a guide to a description of what the concerns are: i.e., what the ultimate objectives of policy are.

Our interpretation of these is that it is the objective to make receipt of health care independent of ability to pay for it but instead to make it equally available to those in 'need.' The quotation marks indicate, of course, that this term has yet to be defined. A further objective is to provide appropriate levels of care at maximum efficiency (i.e., at least social cost).

We hope to show that, once 'need' is defined in an appropriate way, these two broad objectives encompass the entire objective of health policy. For example, concern about geographical equity will be interpreted as concern about relating the availability of resources to 'need' — wherever it may be geographically located. The concern is described as geographical, we suppose, because of a presumption that 'needs' are geographically distributed differently from the distribution of resources. Concern about the secular tendency for health care expenditures to rise may be viewed more relevantly as concerns about income distribution on the one hand and efficiency on the other: since the level of expenditure is the quantity of resources used multiplied by their prices, part of the concern relates to changing factor rewards as the relative prices of factors change; part of the concern relates to the quantity of real resources, whether it is the 'right' amount, effectively deployed; and part relates to the over-all cost, and its rate of growth, in relation to the needs that, at the margin, are being met.

In the next chapter we go a step further. We there argue that, while there may exist an ultimate conflict between the goals of having both an efficient and fair health service, it seems unlikely that Ontario has yet reached the point where some equity must be sacrificed for the sake of efficiency and cost control. The principal basis for this view will be that while the introduction of 'deterrent pricing' controls expenditure but only at the cost of equity, policies that act on prices to consumers are likely to have less impact on expenditure growth (and efficiency) than more direct controls; controls which, moreover, do not conflict with equity objectives. By shifting policy attention further away from the demand for health services and from the mere distribution of inputs towards the *productivity* of the services in improving health, we argue that the interests of both efficiency and equity may mutually be served with detriment to neither.

4
Health measurement in the public interest

Suppose that we had an indicator of health 'need' of the sort mentioned (but not specified) in chapter three. Suppose also that we knew at all times how most effectively to meet the 'need' (so our knowledge would include a knowledge of which procedures were altogether *in*effective at meeting 'need'). Suppose finally that we knew also how to provide these 'need'-meeting procedures at least cost. If these three suppositions were granted, only one outstanding problem of health service management would remain – how large (in terms of resources, or the value of resources used up) the health sector ought to be: a question requiring politicians to evaluate the further effective reduction of health 'needs' relative to the cost of not meeting other kinds of needs in, say, education, housing or private consumption. Given a budget for the health sector, however, the most efficient disposition of resources within the health sector would be readily calculable – provided, of course, that the objective of minimizing 'need' were accepted as 'the' objective for the health sector.

The fulfilment of an objective consisting of the maximum reduction in health 'needs' out of given resources would, it may be plausibly argued, destroy the apparent conflict between efficiency and equity in health care. Equity has usually been interpreted as requiring equal accessibility to health care resources independently of a person's income, class, geographic, etc., status. In practice, this has brought attention to focus upon per capita provision levels in geographical areas. It has also, however, usually been realized that the blind pursuit of such a distribution of resources would be foolish because 'need' varies and it seems manifestly inequitable that areas of high health 'needs' have no more resources per capita than those of low 'needs.' Similarly, the composition of 'need' varies according to demographic and morbidity patterns in different locations and some 'needs' require more, or costlier, or at least different, resources from others.

But it is not merely that the focus of traditional concern about equity upon *input* levels must be modified by considerations of 'need.' A proper interpretation of public concerns in health care provision requires us not to be concerned *at all* with equal input provision but to focus, instead, upon *outcomes,* or the impact that resources may have upon 'need.' If we so allocated our health care resources that the maximum reduction in 'need' were obtained then we would *not* observe equal input provision per capita. Indeed, if we sought from this position to make the input distribution more equal it would inevitably follow that we would *increase the amount of unmet 'need' in society.*

There is, however, a notion of equality, of a sort, embodied in the pursuit of the maximum reduction of 'need.' This notion flows from a characteristic of the efficient reduction of 'need,' namely that the ratio of a unit of reduction in measured 'need' to its cost should everywhere (and for everyone) be equal. If we could (which we often cannot) identify social cost with public expenditure in the health sector, then we could alternatively describe this equality condition as requiring an equal reduction in 'need' per marginal dollar of public spending in each area, for each client group, etc.

Clearly, this approach would imply that only effective regimes of care, prevention, or cure, would be provided. Individuals in 'need' but for whom no effective regime currently existed would remain no less in 'need.' This is not the harsh implication of a policy of utilizing only productive regimes in a health sector of unyielding rationality, but is a direct implication of a moral commitment to making the greatest possible reduction in 'need': wasting resources in procedures that have no effect means denying them to other patients who would benefit.

The policy of maximum 'need' reduction thus encompasses both efficiency and equity arguments and enables us – in principle at least – to escape the dilemma noted in the first section of chapter three. But that section, which was quite traditional in its approach, based its efficiency arguments upon individual willingness to pay. Later in that chapter we argued that Ontario policy should probably not be based upon willingness to pay. The main reason put there was that the prevailing value judgment seems to be that health resource allocation should be based upon whether or not individuals are in 'need,' or at risk. To this we may add that it is extremely difficult to identify willingness to pay without actually having people pay. But since Ontario does not currently have *marginal* user prices for health care consumers (which are the relevant ones for efficiency in the willingness-to-pay model) and neither is there any serious pressure for their introduction, there appears no valid basis either in principle or practice for willingness to pay to be a principle for guiding allocation. Instead we have patients' 'needs' determined, once they come into contact with the system, by the medical profession. Within the sanctity of the doctor-patient relationship and behind the protective professional screen of clinical freedom, both what a patient 'needs' and what he shall receive are determined.

The system, we therefore argue, is already based upon an interpretation of 'need' – an interpretation that traditional medical training makes medical professionals feel to be (and with much legitimacy) a natural and central part of clinical practice.

Moreover, since the quotation marks around need, indicating its lack of a definition, must by now be becoming as much an irritation to the reader as they are an inconvenience to the author, it is time for the definition. It is two-fold. A need for health care exists when: (*a*) the potential for *avoidance* of reductions in health status exists (prevention and some care) (*b*) the potential for *improvements* in health status above the level it would otherwise be exists (cure and some care).

These definitions have some characteristics lacking in others that have been commonly put (for a review, see Culyer, 1976, chap. 2). First, the need for a service is related to what that service may *accomplish* in terms of the well-being of the patient. Second, the need is not absolute: the fact that a potential may exist does not imply that it must be realized, for realizing a potential uses up resources that could have been devoted to other desired ends, and a balance must be struck. Third, and as we shall shortly see in great detail, the notion of health status is very heavily endowed with value-judgments whose nature must be explored, while the notion of potential is primarily a technical concept concerning the effectiveness of procedures of prevention, care, or cure.

Fourth, and a point which appears to be a weakness of the definition, is that it seems to imply that where there is no potential (perhaps because there is no currently available and effective procedure) there is also no need. Plainly, it is not meaningless to speak, say, of someone needing a treatment that does not yet exist. But this limitation is more apparent than real, for the 'potential' now attaches itself by implication to the prospects for *research* rather than prevention, care, or cure. That is, those who may need non-existent 'treatments' are best seen as needing the results of successfully prosecuted research. This has the great advantage of focusing policy thinking in the right direction, and hopefully focusing clinical practice that way too, for it is well known that we commonly give expensive but ineffective treatments to those who are undoubtedly in need of the results of research, but can scarcely be said to be in need of *ineffective* treatments![1]

The remainder of this chapter is devoted to an analysis of the essential logic of health status measurement to show precisely where there is a need for value judgments and to identify clearly the separate boxes into which the analysis of outputs and the analysis of inputs (their potential for influencing outputs) should be seen to fit.

HEALTH OUTPUT AND HEALTH CARE PRODUCTION

A conceptual approach which embodies the above, which encompasses both the macro kind of measure as well as the micro measures discussed in chapter two and, moreover, which enables us clearly to distinguish inputs and outputs, is set out in the remainder of this chapter in terms of the 'political economy' of health measures developed in Culyer, Lavers, and Williams (1971).

Beginning at the highest level of all we consider health vis-à-vis other publicly provided or subsidized services. (The framework could be readily extended to include choice concerning the choice of the public sector as a whole vis-à-vis the private sector.) We assume that a rational choice will be based upon the *outputs* of public policies (for some practical reasons why politicians may actually try to behave this way with the limited information available to them, and for a model in which such behaviour is central, see Breton, 1974).

In Figure 2, the axes measure (on a ratio, or at least an interval, scale)[2] the output of the health services and the output of educational institutions: outputs which we may, for the moment, think of in terms of health status on the one hand and perhaps some weighted combination of measures of cognitive, affective, and psychomotor development on the other (see Greenberg 1974 a, b for further development). The simplifying assumptions of two sectors only, each with a single output, are made for expository simplicity. With a given budget and given technologies we suppose that in any decision period resources devoted to output in one sector can be transferred to producing output in the other only at increasing marginal (opportunity) cost as shown by the transformation locus *EaH*: the decision-makers may choose a maximum of *OE* education *or OH* health or some combination lying along *EaH*.

---

1 Another kind of need is also excluded by the definition: the care and comfort which, it may be felt, ought to go to certain dependent groups and terminal cases. Plainly such persons may be in need in a variety of important ways. What they do not typically need, however, is medical care. To the extent that they do not meet our twin definitions, whatever they need it is not medical care.
2 See below at pp. 71-2 for more discussion.

Figure 2

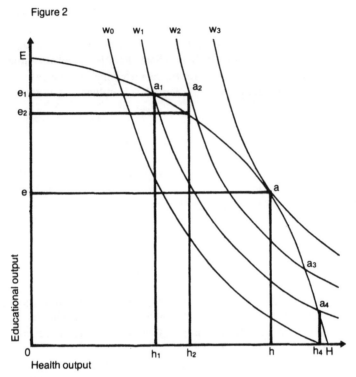

We now suppose that the political decision-makers have some preference function characterized by the concave (from above) indifference curves $W_0, ..., W_3$. These may be viewed as determined by some set of (here unspecified) factors such as manifesto commitment, party or personal philosophy, electoral pressures, and so on. Clearly the rational fully-informed decision-maker will locate at a, implying outputs of Oe education and Oh health.

The framework of Figure 2 gives us the opportunity for an explicit discussion of two central themes in this book: (a) the notion of 'need,' (b) the immense information requirement which, at present, make even this stylized model largely unoperational. We discuss each in turn.

Output and 'need'
Special interest groups are frequently successful in persuading governments to behave as though inputs were outputs. Breton (1974) discusses an example where the government seeks to maximize the output of a public service such as police protection subject to a budget constraint *and* a prescribed utilization of manpower. More generally, one could model a political choice between rates of

output produced using inputs and one (or more) of the rates of input utilization as though it itself were an output.

Because of the pressure on governments, it is not necessarily irrational for them to consider inputs as though they were outputs, or to treat particular quotas of input utilization as exogenously given. Nevertheless, for our purposes it is convenient to set aside such phenomena – which may be extremely important features of analyses purporting to *explain* government behaviour -- in order to focus exclusively on 'public interest' dimensions, which we take, following the discussion of chapter three, to be concerned with ultimate outputs. Certainly, high-minded discussions of need are correct in viewing inputs as *policy instruments,* as means to the ultimate ends that are needed, *viz.,* better health, a better educated citizenry, etc.

In this context, our analysis immediately suggests the inappropriateness of needs expressed as absolutes or *targets.* Suppose, for example, that in some previous time period a_1 had been chosen as the optimal combination of E and H, *viz.,* current resources are allocated so as to maintain levels Oe_1 education and Oh_1 health. Suppose, moreover, that political decision-makers asserted that really Oh_2 health were needed, in the sense that it was a target aimed at. The implied target is located at a_2 which, given the budget, the technical possibilities, and a commitment to Oe_1 education, is, under the circumstances, quite unattainable. *Insistence* on Oh_2 health would imply a switch of resources, giving only Oe_2 education. A target which ignores the necessary costs of getting there is plainly mere rhetoric, of use only to politicians when window-dressing, or to social reformers in particular areas who are not in the unhappy position of having to count the cost of going without public service in areas other than those they are concerned with. This view of need is a less extreme form of the technocratic concept of need as exemplified by Cohen (1968): 'we are still far from assuring every American the right to the best health care that modern medical science makes possible.' By definition, modern medical science can possibly take us to *OH.* This is the full potential reduction in need: with an implied distribution of resources between E and *H* that no one in their right minds, or who cared to think a little about the problem of public decision-making, would seriously entertain for one moment.

Plainly, a socially relevant notion of need must therefore at once be both *relative* and *marginal*: relative to the other good things which must be sacrificed and marginal in that the more we succeed in meeting need in one field, the less urgent (again relative to other needs or demands) further degrees of success become. Fortunately, if our characterization of public decision-makers' preferences in Figure 2 is approximately correct, there is no danger of their actually *behaving* as if need were not relative and marginal (regardless of what they may actually say). Moreover, the evidence points overwhelmingly to the plausibility of our assumption. (For further dissection of need see Williams, 1974b).

There is, however, no immediate prospect of this highly aggregative use of measures of need in public decision-making. The value of the analysis lies rather, on the one hand, in its enabling us quite easily to dismiss some of the rhetoric of social indicators propaganda as unhelpful and, on the other, in providing a decision-theoretic framework for more detailed analysis of health status measures that have some prospect of being helpful in the not-too-distant future. These developments consist in devising measures that correspond to some of the key dimensions and parameters of Figure 2 and, in particular, the measurement of health status (corresponding to H in the figure) and its relationship to the inputs that are believed to affect it: the measurement of output and the production function.

Output and production

As we shall see in the next chapter, a useful geometrical expository device relates the various components of health status measure so as to enable the calculation of a single measure (whether single or multiple measures are to be preferred is also discussed in chapter five).

Health status is to be defined in terms of individuals' ability to function in society independently and without pain or anxiety. This is, of course, to be sharply distinguished from what is done in a diagnostic situation where the object is to attach a clinical label to a patient's condition which in turn is helpful in assigning treatments and making prognoses, though clinical notions of urgency and treatment cannot altogether escape a social assessment of the kind implied here. Our emphasis, however, is upon the social significance of disease and handicapping conditions: a clinical condition, if such exists, that has no, or entirely trivial, consequences in terms of functional impairment, pain, and anxiety, and, moreover, has no prospect of developing into such a condition, is, in our view, socially unimportant. For *illustrative* purposes in this chapter, we suppose there to be only two relevant dimensions in a measure of ill-health, which we shall make the personal characteristics 'painfulness' and 'restriction of activity.' For those who prefer to think in more aggregate terms, we could have chosen, say, 'GP consultations per year' as a crude morbidity indicator, and 'perinatal mortality rate,' though these would not have raised *all* of the basic issues we must confront with the more micro dimensions we have chosen. Moreover, they suffer from disadvantages noted earlier. In particular, GP consultations are institutionally not community based, while perinatal mortality is a crude measure of health status whose chief virtue appears to be that it is believed to be more closely related to the quality of health care received than are other kinds of mortality.

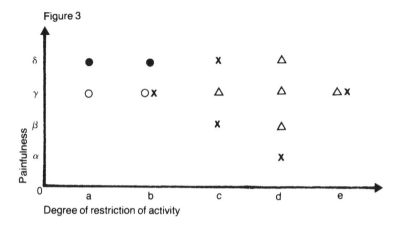

Figure 3

The first step is to experiment with simple standardized *descriptions* of painfulness and of the degree to which activity is restricted, to see if there is any consensus among medical personnel (or patients, or some other set of appropriate experts) as to how painful and how restricting particular conditions are, using these descriptive categories (see Figure 3). α, β, γ, and δ are simple descriptive statements concerned with painfulness (such as 'mildly uncomfort-able,' 'very uncomfortable,' 'extremely painful,' etc.). a, b, c, d, and e are simple descriptive statements concerned with restriction of activity (such as light work only, confined to house and immediate vicinity, confined to house, confined to bedroom, confined to bed, etc.). Many of the actual categories used in experiments and case-studies are described in some detail in the next chapter. 0, x, and Δ each refer to different medical conditions or different combinations of medical conditions. For example, the medical condition Δ in Figure 3 is regarded by one observer as involving, for a patient suffering from it, degrees of painfulness and restricted activity described by the statements γ and d respectively. Of the other four observers who place condition Δ in the 'painfulness-restricted activity' space, two agree with the statement of the first observer on painfulness (but categorize the degree of restricted activity by statements c and e) and two agree with the statement of the first observer on activity restriction (but regard associated painfulness as being better described by statements β and δ). Each 0 plotted on Figure 3 represents one expert's assessment of the most appropriate description of that condition in the categories offered (e.g., one says a, δ; another says a, γ; another says b, δ and yet another b, γ). Similarly each x represents corresponding judgments by other experts of the most appropriate descriptions of those conditions. The specifica-tion of medical conditions may, of course, have reference to age, social class, and other attributes, and the degree of articulation would have to be such that

Figure 4

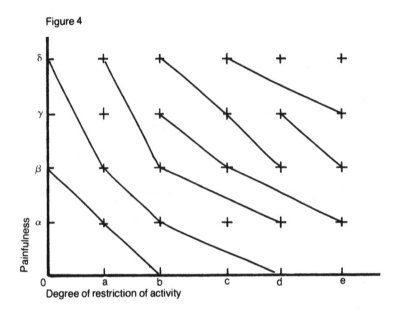

Degree of restriction of activity

patients suffering from each condition formed a relatively homogeneous group. If there is any consistency in these judgments (as there is in 0 and △ in the example) some 'norm' will be indicated as the standard description for that condition; where no consensus exists (as with x in the example) it is likely that the condition under study needs to be more closely specified.

However, supposing that we had each condition clearly ascribed to a pain category (α, β, γ, etc.) and a restricted-activity category (a, b, c, etc.), the next stage consists in finding some way of combining the two dimensions in order to make an over-all appraisal of a patient's condition, or to compare his with another's. As we shall see in chapter five there are many ways in which this can be, and has been, done. Here we illustrate by making pairwise comparisons (e.g., is the combination a better or worse than the combination βc?). This pairwise comparison is essentially a social judgment and should be recognized as such. This first evaluative step is set out diagrammatically in Figure 4. Each combination of a pain category (α,β,γ, etc.) and a restricted-activity category (a, b, c, etc.) is compared, and those that are regarded as approximately equivalent (in terms of social-humanitarian benefit of avoiding them) are linked together by contour lines as indicated. In the example shown, the combinations (β, 0); (α, a); and (0, b) are equivalent to each other, but better than (γ, 0) and (0, c) (which may be equivalent to each other). Those in turn are better than the next group of equivalents (β, a), (a, b), and (0, d), and so on.

Despite the fact that describing the intensity of pain is notoriously difficult and interpersonal comparisons are bound to be rather arbitrary, for example, because of varying thresholds of pain, medical personnel can and do make such comparisons between stages and classes of condition, and such comparisons already have to be assimilated into judgments about 'acceptable' degress of physical disability and pain at the diagnostic and therapeutic level when determing courses of treatment.

The next stage (again involving value judgments) consists in ascribing numbers to the contours. Since it is intended to use these numbers as the measure of health status they must typically represent more than a mere ordering: they should represent a measure of ill-health on a ratio scale (where only the unit of measurement is arbitrary), or at least on an interval scale (where the origin as well as the unit is arbitrary). The former enables us to make statements like 'contour a is five times worse than contour b' and 'the move from contour c to contour d is twice as bad as the move from contour a to contour b.' The latter enables only the second kind of comparison.

As introductory examples of the kind of uses to which these basic ideas may be put, two illustrations follow: first a cost-effectiveness application; second measurement of community health status.

In cost-effectiveness analysis of health procedures, it is well known that we should be sure we are costing alternative ways of doing essentially the same thing – in our case, effecting a health improvement. This plainly requires us to consider the duration of periods of ill-health. In Figure 5 we start at time O, when the condition in question is diagnosed. In the illustrative example the first two weeks are spent in further observation and waiting for therapeutic facilities to become available.

The prognosis without treatment (or with the best treatment other than that under consideration) is represented by the broken line and may be described as a steady deterioration from approximately week 7, until death in week 12 (which is here assumed to be the worst possible state, being assigned the score 10). This would be the standard prediction for this class of case. The average expectation of life for a person of that age/sex, etc. is represented as $(N + M)$ which may be rather large if necessary (e.g., 50 years).

The prognosis with treatment is represented by the solid line, and may be described as two weeks of severe restriction of activity (in the pre-operative, operative, and immediate post-operative phases) plus, possibly, considerable pain, with a steady improvement in condition during the ensuring 3 weeks, a convalescent phase from weeks 7 to 9, and a further 2 weeks taking it easy in a normal environment, after which the patient is completely normal.

The total impact on health status (representing the 'effectiveness' of this treatment) would be the area under the dotted line minus the area under the

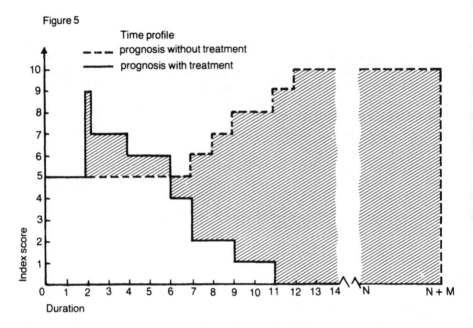

Figure 5

Time profile
- - - prognosis without treatment
——— prognosis with treatment

solid line – in net terms the large shaded area less the small one. This is the *potential for improvement* identified above at p. 46. This particular example would be a highly effective treatment if applied to people with long life expectancy, less so for those having a shorter life expectancy. Both of the time profiles used would be derived from statistical analyses of clinical results, or experimental data if the former were lacking. A further sophistication which could be introduced if necessary would be to apply a discounting factor which would give less weight to future states of health compared with present states, and hence reflect the greater weight people seem to attach to the 'here and now' rather than to more distant prospects. In this way the use of the measure would serve to narrow the area of uncertainty about the consequences of alternative patterns of resource allocation.

As a measure of a community's or a region's health status the same categories could be used as a basis for a large-scale statistical survey, the object of which would be to measure both the index score and the duration of the various conditions affecting the population. Repeated periodically throughout the year (to allow for seasonal fluctuations) and from year to year (to establish trends) this would provide the kind of information required as a contribution to general social indicators, and would be free of many of the defects inherent in medical record-based statistics. In particular, it would include cases where people had not presented themselves for treatment, or where those giving treatment were unaware of the patient's condition between episodes of treatment.[3]

The cost-effectiveness illustration is an example of one kind of 'production function' study using an outcome measure to aid in the choice of technique. We shall confront several empirical examples of such analyses in later chapters. Less well-developed is more aggregate work related to the effects of a broad set of resources, including environmental factors, upon the health status of groups of people (for example, geographical groups).

Such studies might, depending on their purpose, postulate either a single community health index or a vector of health attributes as a function of a vector of independent variables (e.g., hospital beds per population, doctors, distance from health facilities, weather, housing conditions). Alternatively, the effects of such independent variables on the probability of transition from one health state to another might be measured.

In their nature, such aggregate 'production functions' must be less refined than those whose use is principally seen at the micro level, but they can provide broad guidelines as to the productivity of health spending in different regions or for different client groups and hence aid in the objective of minimizing health needs.

The distinction between these two kinds of use of health status measures is important and will become particularly significant when we come to discuss in later chapters the steps that might be taken in Ontario. Lest anyone should be tempted to suppose that what is being advocated is a counsel of perfection, it is as well to emphasize now that in both these uses (broad or macro and specific or micro) practicalities are going to compel a high degree of selectivity.

In particular, the measurement of community health status is a *general* measure, of value chiefly because it draws attention to apparent 'problems,' just as currently, we can use perinatal mortality data in the province to identify areas where there seems to be a problem. Clearly, 'doing' something about it requires more detailed and specific investigation of the 'causes,' of ways of reducing the rate and their costs. So it is with the general health status measure. We will want, typically, to identify the health status of particular client groups such as children, industrial workers, the elderly. Once an apparent anomaly is identified we have to become much more specific and that is where detailed analysis of

3 An extremely useful review of the common features of index construction, given the basic units in which it is to be measured, is Torrance (1976) where he shows that they may all be reduced to a basic model related to aggregation across individuals' index scores, individuals' disease states, and through time. Our concern here, and in the next chapter, however, is chiefly with the derivation of the basic index score itself.

input-output relationships again comes in. There is no question that *every* program needs detailed evaluation. The general measure gives two useful general pieces of information – it enables the development of rules of thumb for general revenue allocation (which are bound to be approximate) and it enables the identification of specific issues warranting detailed attention. The criteria for selecting such specific areas might include: (*a*) the fact that the health status measure for a particular area, client group, etc., shows a marked deviation from the norm, (*b*) the judgment that a particular area, client group, etc. is of some special importance, (*c*) the fact that the particular problem is thought to cause heavy costs, (*d*) the fact that a particular program is extremely costly and resource savings are urgently wanted, (*e*) the fact that the technology for dealing with the problem is well understood and is affective, and (*f*) the fact that a new and effective technology has recently become available for a particular problem. This list is not, of course, exhaustive.

At the micro level illustrated by our cost-effectiveness example, again the idea is not that *all* programs should be put through their paces in this way. Aside from the fact that this would not be possible anyway since the natural history of many illness is too imperfectly understood, such a comprehensive analytical assault would clog the system hopelessly. Two micro uses of health status measure are likely on a selective basis, to be most practicable. The first is in clinical research concerned with effectiveness – the effective impact of preventive or curative measures upon health status. This area of the 'micro-production function' of health in the health services (which are not, of course, the only inputs) is arguably the single most important area for research even though in the present book we pay it relatively little attention (see Culyer, 1976). In such studies, an appropriate index of outcome is essential. And it is not necessarily to be expected that health services are in all (or even most) cases the most effective way of meeting health needs. The second is in cost-effectiveness studies. The criteria for selecting programs or procedures for an efficiency study are essentially the six outlined above. In particular, it should be noted that there is very little point in an efficiency study if any one or more of the following is the case: (*a*) there are no substantially different alternative procedures to choose from, (*b*) the technology of care of the alternative has no firmly agreed base, (*c*) the effectiveness of the technologies is unknown. Each of these precludes the *possibility* of conducting the analysis.

Whatever the purpose to which these techniques are applied, however, health status measurement normally involves one in implicitly or explicitly going through the analytical stages outlined above. As we have seen, some of the issues involved are of a technical kind (some of which are, in turn, medical in nature) but others crucially concern values. Even if we draw back from high-level decisions about whether to meet further needs, value judgments are inescapably embodied in health status index construction. Because they are so crucial, and because they do not always receive the explicit attention they deserve, the whole of the next chapter is devoted to their discussion. The opportunity is also taken there to show how actual measures have been constructed by different researchers.

5

Trade-offs and values
in health measures

In chapter four, we saw that health status measurement necessarily involves making value judgments. Of course, other kinds of judgment are also required. In this chapter, however, we focus on value judgments and, in particular, those relating to trade-offs between components of an index. In summary, the value judgments necessarily embodied in a health status measure that is for use in planning decisions are the following: 1. a choice of dimensions for the measure; 2. a set of choices concerning how the dimensions are to be traded off one against the other – and how these relative trade-offs are to change (*viz.*, along a given health status contour); 3. a set of choices concerning how numbers are to be assigned to the health status contours identified in (2); 4. a set of choices concerning the correspondence between the numbers (or changes in the numbers) of (3) and their pecuniary equivalents (or their value relative to non-health outputs); 5. having made the benefits commensurable with the cost of effecting them (in step 4) the final value judgment concerns a rejection of policies for whom the value of benefits falls short of the costs. It is the basic value judgment to which an economic approach commits us: namely that a service should be provided only if its social benefits exceed its social costs.[1]

In addition, other value judgments may also be introduced by some of the techniques used to derive the values. One such as we shall see, concerns attitudes to risk. As we shall see, few studies have to date succeeded in working through

---

1 And even this is only a necessary, not a sufficient, condition for the efficiency of a policy.

all of these steps. Such is only to be expected in a field which remains, at the moment, largely experimental. We shall also find that some methods combine what we have here itemized as separate value steps (for example, (2) and (3) are often combined, as when numbers are directly assigned to combinations of function levels: so are (2), (3), and (4), as when 'output' is treated as the contribution to production of an individual restored to work). The value of identifying these separately derives from the possibility that it will be felt that different arbiters of value are preferred at each stage and also from the fact that, depending on the uses to which the index is to be put, not all successive stages need to be gone through.

A variety of meanings attaches to the word 'value' and it is therefore as well to be aware of its connotations in our present context. The term will be used in three senses here. In the first use it has its usual ethical content in that 'value judgments' express a judgment about what is ethically to be desired (what is desirable). A second sense is the usual sociological/psychological sense, where it refers to those ends or means that an individual desires (what is desired). Values in this sense describe an individual's preferences. Values in the former sense refer to those entities that are regarded (by someone) as *desirable:* ethical imperatives. Thus he may desire that which he also regards as undesirable. The third sense is the most frequent sense used in economics, which derives from the second, but refers to marginal values, or the relative desire an individual has for a little more of this relative to that. 'Value' will be used in each of these senses in the present chapter and the context of its use should make clear which meaning is implied in each case.

In the remainder of this chapter, we consider each of the first three value judgments itemized above and explore how the literature has (sometimes only implicitly) treated them. The first three judgments inhere in almost all health status measures.

CHOICE OF DIMENSIONS

Not all the judgments that have to be made are value judgments. This is important to note since the qualifications that persons are required to have to make judgments of fact, or judgments about technology, need not be the same as the qualifications they are required to have to make judgments of value. Such an observation may appear jejune and uncontroversial. Nevertheless, at least one distinguished economist would dissent from it:

My personal feeling is that the value judgments made by economists are, by and large, better than those made by non-economists! ... My assertion about value judgments is not as arrogant as it sounds. For one thing, it applies only to the sort of value judgments involved in public investment decisions, and even here does not apply to all of them ... The point is simply that the people who are experienced at systematic thinking about a problem are usually those who make the best judgments about it. Thus, whatever their theory of aesthetics, most people are prepared in practice to accept the judgment of an art critic about the merits of a painting. (Turvey, 1963, 96)

Unfortunately it is not clear from this, nor from the example (not quoted) that Turvey gives, which value judgments actually are best made by economists or, more generally, by 'experts.' Nor is it clear why 'systematic thinking' (presumably referring to the kind of thoughts characteristic of economists) is conducive to 'good' value judgments – though we may readily concede that economists (or any systematic thinkers) may be quite adept at distinguishing value judgments from other kinds of judgment. Indeed, such distinctions are what we may reasonably expect from systematic thought of any kind.

One distinquished sociologist had made the point very forcibly with regard to the autonomy of the medical profession:

There is a real danger of a new tyranny which sincerely expresses itself in the language of humanitarianism and which imposes its own values on others for what it sees to be their own good ... [We should be concerned with] delineating the question of what is expertise and what concealed class morality, and what is actual performance rather than unrealizable ethical intent ... It is my own opinion that the professions' role in a free society should be limited to contributing the technical information men need to make their own decisions on the basis of their own values. When he preempts the authority to direct, even constrain men's decisions on the basis of his own values, the professional is no longer an expert but rather a member of a new privileged class disguised as an expert. (Freidson, 1970, 381-2)

Many of the value judgments we shall discuss in the present chapter are arguably 'best' (i.e., legitimately) made by non-experts – in particular by non-economists *and* by non-physicians. As far as choice of dimensions is concerned, however, an important part of the selection can be made quite independently of value judgments: the judgments that are required are of quite different kinds.

Some of these points can be illustrated from the well-worked territory of programs designed to help the elderly. The objectives of such programs are commonly defined in rather broad terms such as social integration (to reduce social isolation of the elderly within the community); self-dependence (to preserve identity and independence of the elderly); physical well-being (Algie, 1972). These aspirations are, of course, essential value judgments and, although the experience of social workers may be helpful in identifying different ways of, say, integrating such people, and that of economists in costing alternative procedures, the value systems that imply that these dimensions are, or should be, the objectives of policy do not necessarily emanate from, or only from, such professional groups.

By contrast, from the *circumstances* of the case it may sometimes be inferred that some specific dimensions are more relevant than others. Thus, a program where the physical abilities of elderly persons in residential homes is judged important would not normally be concerned with ability to cook, do shopping, or do carpet cleaning because such tasks are not performed by such persons (Wright, 1974). The *purpose* of the exercise likewise may suggest some measures of ability as being more relevant than others: ability to cut toenails may be an important component in an indicator of the need for chiropody services, but there may be superior indicators measuring the impact of a program on patients' general ability to manage for themselves: ability to dress measures ability to grasp and manipulate small objects (zips, buttons, etc.), to bend and stretch, etc. Clearly, there may also exist correlations between abilities enabling some to be eliminated as redundant in an index of general physical well-being.

A more macrosocial example of technical choice concerns that between use of infant mortality rates (deaths within one year of live-born infants per 1000 live born) as against perinatal mortality rates (still births and deaths under one week of age) or neo-natal mortality rates (deaths of infants under four weeks of age). The latter two rates are more related to medical care provision than the former, because other social and economic factors (such as housing, income) have important influences. Thus, if the focus of interest is the effectiveness of medical services, peri-natal mortality is a more interesting statistic than infant mortality.

It is sometimes the case that a lexicographic ordering of characteristics adequately scales a continuum of sickness or disability which obviates the necessity for trading-off the individual characteristics. For example, if individuals having difficulty with feeding also have difficulty with continence, ambulation, dressing, and bathing; individuals having difficulty with continence also have difficulty with ambulation, dressing, and bathing, etc., then for the above five characteristics each dichotomized into difficulty/no difficulty states, the potential 2^5 (= 32) combinations can be collapsed into 6 categories of ordinarily ranked degrees of dependence as indicated in Table 3. The scale is

TABLE 3

Guttman scale of patient dependence

Degree of dependence	Feeding	Continence	Ambulation	Dressing	Bathing
1	no	no	no	no	no
2	no	no	no	no	yes
3	no	no	no	yes	yes
4	no	no	yes	yes	yes
5	no	yes	yes	yes	yes
6	yes	yes	yes	yes	yes

termed a Guttman scale (after Guttman, 1944) and whether it is possible or useful depends, of course, in part on the combinations of patient states that are actually observed. Thus, if as many patients have (yes, no, no, no, no,) as (no, no, no, no, yes) the scale will not be of much help. The better the 'fit' in this sense the more perfect the scale type. How perfect one requires it to be is a matter largely of judgment.

There exist methods of adjusting characteristics and the cut-off points which determine whether a 'yes' or a 'no' answer is recorded, which maximize the 'perfection' of the Guttman scale (Tenhouten, 1969) and which were utilized by Skinner and Yett (1973) to derive a Guttman scale of debility for patients needing skilled nursing care in a cost study of nursing homes. The technique, where applicable, has an obvious use as an ordinal indicator of 'need.' Skinner and Yett (1973) were able to identify the distribution of patients by dependence and institution as in Table 4.

It should be noted that the categories used by Skinner and Yett were those developed by Katz *et al.* (1963) in devising their index of activities of daily living for elderly persons with fracture of the hip. This pioneering work used dichotomous yes/no categories and devised an ordinal index as follows: A: independence in feeding, continence, transferring, going to toilet, dressing, and bathing; B: independent in all but one of these functions; C: independent in all but bathing and one additional function; D: independent in all but bathing, dressing, and one additional function; E: independent in all but bathing, dressing, going to toilet, and one additional function; F: independent in all but bathing, dressing, going to toilet, transferring, and one additional function; G: dependent in all six functions; 'other': dependent in at least two functions, but not classifiable as C, D, E, or F.

In the further sample of 1001 old persons (not necessarily with fracture of the hip) only 4 percent fell into the 'other' category and it seems clear that this

TABLE 4

Percentage distribution of 21,036 patients by degree of dependence

Location	Degree of dependence					
	1	2	3	4	5	6
Nursing homes	14.9	12.0	24.5	12.2	12.1	24.3
Long-term hospital	23.0	10.3	19.1	13.5	12.8	21.3
Long-term unit in general hospital	23.0	10.8	16.2	17.3	12.6	20.1

SOURCE: Skinner and Yett (1973, 75)

procedure is an extremely effective one for these categories in deriving an ordinal index. The dichotomous nature of the units of measuring ability to function, however, has been criticized by several authors (Wright, 1974, and references there) and makes the approach inappropriate where focus is upon degrees of dependency of a subtler kind. Its usefulness has been proved, however, in prognosis where it enables the avoidance of prolonged therapeutic efforts whose outcome, as measured by the index, is unlikely to be successful.

Another statistical technique that has been used is factor analysis. Levine and Yett (1973) used this in order to reduce a large number of regional indicators of health status, environment and socio-economic conditions into a more manageable number of variables (four in their case). The essence of the procedure is to hypothesize that there exists some variable, health status, that is a function of a smaller set of unobservable *factors* which underly the 63 available indicators. The idea is to derive weights or 'loadings' based on the correlation between observed variables such that the factors are uncorrelated with one another while the loadings are regression coefficients of factors that explain a high proportion of the variance of the jth observed indicator. By observing the factor with the highest loading for each observed variable, the latter may then be grouped into clusters that (one hopes) make sense (e.g., all observed variables concerning income have relatively high loadings on one factor). For each cluster a composite index is then derived statistically and these can be related to socio-demographic and economic variables.

This technique has been of use in some areas (e.g., psychology) where there is little theory available to determine which variables are or ought to be relevant, and there may be some use for it in *positive* applications in the health territory, for example, in ascertaining what variables or groups of variables have greatest impact on morbidity. Since, however, nothing of normative import can be inferred from an analysis making no normative assumptions and since normative issues largely predominate in status measurement (What is 'need'? Is that disability 'worse' than this one? Is a sick child 'worth' higher priority than an equally sick adult?) we propose no further discussions of factor analysis here. The procedure would seem *not* to be appropriate for the purpose conceived for it by Levine and Yett: namely to identify areas whose health status is low. Low health status is a policy issue that is not decidable on grounds of correlation alone. And this is quite aside from the inherent abstruseness of a technique, which is scarcely likely to commend itself for this if no other reason to the political masters, administrative managers, and clinical practitioners in health services. This must especially be the case since nobody is proposing that health indicators or indexes should wholly *supplant* professional, political, and administrative judgment. The aim is to *supplement* these informal judgments in order to make social judgments more systematically. It therefore follows that too high a degree of sophistication, producing results that are hard to interpret, is absolutely to be avoided.

We thus find that choice of the dimensions of an index is partly a question of values, of interpreting the specific objects of policy, and partly a technical question, concerning valid, reliable, economical, and reproducible methods of measuring the objects. Just as persons who may legitimately be thought to have a claim on the right to formulate objects of policy (e.g., the elderly, the representatives of those financing the program) may have little competence in deciding those matters we have described as 'technical,' so those with this latter competence are not necessarily those regarded as having a legitimate right to decide objectives, or trade-offs.

TRADING-OFF DIMENSIONS

For evaluative purposes, the necessity for trade-offs will normally be inescapable even to identify only the qualitative *direction of change* in an individual's or a group's condition. Figure 6 shows the results reported in McDowell and Martini (n.d.) of before-after (steroid treatment) interviews with a patient suffering from Crohn's disease. The patient was presented with a set of statements describing deviations from 'normal' behaviour and asked which of the statements described her current situation. The questionnaire in this instance covered twelve aspects of everyday living (excluding work since the patients were working neither before nor afterwards) with sleeping and eating combined in the same category. As the figure reveals, the number of 'yes' responses had increased in one dimension, not changed in two, and had fallen in the remainder. Whether or not the steroid treatment is regarded *over-all* as beneficial (and ignoring longer-term developments and the persistence of the post-treatment health status) clearly depends

Figure 6
Case of Crohn's Disease before and after alteration of medication

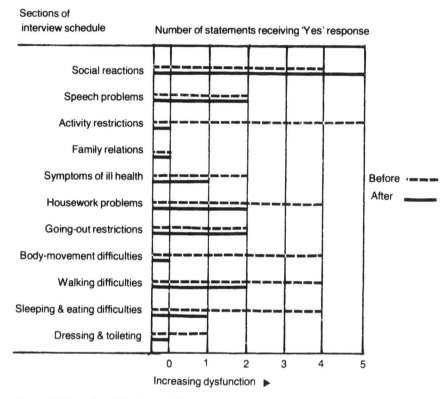

Source: McDowell and Martin (n.d.16).

upon the relative weighting given to the deterioration in social reactions relative to the improvements in activity, etc.

Precisely the same weighting problem arises in connection with geographical comparisons between areas and with longitudinal trends where an over-all view is required, regardless of whether it is related to procedures, environment changes or medical interventions.

Figure 7 shows a scatter of the crude death rate and perinatal death rates for Ontario counties in 1973. These two indicators have commonly been used to compare areas. Taking these two indicators alone, and assuming that lower crude death rates are a 'good thing' and, likewise, low perinatal deaths (not transparently obvious propositions however: the crude death rate should be

Figure 7
Crude death rate and perinatal death rate by county in Ontario, 1973

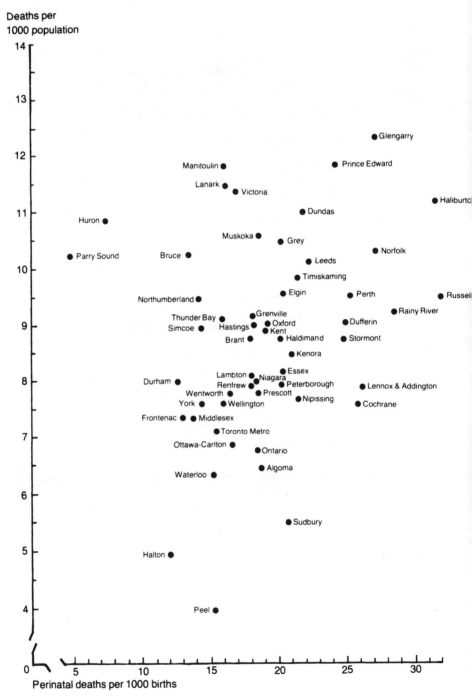

Deaths per
1000 population

Perinatal deaths per 1000 births

adjusted at least for age and sex compositions of the population, while low perinatal mortality may imply a higher prevalence of serious handicap), one tentatively infers that Halton and Peel were 'healthier' than Glengarry and Haliburton. Northeast/southwest comparisons (in the figure) are easy and (granted the assumptions) unambiguous. But what of Parry Sound compared with Sudbury, Durham against Metropolitan Toronto, or Manitoulin against Russell? These comparisons require *weights* to be placed on the dimensions if an over-all judgment is to be made. Note that we are not at this stage attempting to explain or account for these differences in terms of a 'production function' of the sort discussed in chapter four. Rather the concern is with making interregional comparisons of over-all health status.

Miller (1970) identifies essentially the same problem in ranking the social impact of various diseases, where the ranking is quite different depending on whether inpatient days, outpatient visits, or deaths is used and, hence, quite different priorities for program expenditures are implied.

Miller developed the 'Q index' for the US Indian Health Service, which is proposed as just one tool for management in deciding program priorities, and which combined consideration of mortality and morbidity into a single index:

$$Q = (M_i/M_a)DP + (274A + 91.3B)/N,$$

where M_i = age- and sex-adjusted mortality rate of the Indian population; M_a = age- and sex-adjusted mortality rate of the total US population; D = crude mortality rate of Indian population; P = years of life lost because of premature death in the Indian population *(viz.,* the difference between average age of death among Indians and among US population as a whole); A = hospital days in Indian population; B = outpatient visits in Indian population; N = Indian population.

The Q index is clearly a *relative* concept measuring Indian health status relative to that of the US population as a whole though, as Chen (1973) pointed out, it is odd that the morbidity elements (A and B) are not made relative. Indeed, Chen made a number of suggestions for improving this index which we will briefly look at below. Here let us pause to note some of the weights that are applied in the Q index. First, A and B are weighted to convert them to years per 100,000 population with 3 outpatient visits equated in time to one hospital day (since it takes the average Indian one-third of a day to obtain outpatient care, including travel time). The implication of this is that, for a given disease (if the Q index is computed by disease category) the amount of time spent receiving care is the only relevant distinguishing characteristic. The fact (if it *is* a fact!) that hospitalized cases may be more serious cases than outpatient cases is not given weight. It may, of course, be replied that the idea of the Q index is to use currently available data only and to keep the index as straightforward as possible. Against this one might argue that it is no more complex conceptually or practically to weight A and B according to some judgments of their relative seriousness than it is to find out how much more time the one uses up relative to the other.

Second, the simple addition of the mortality and the morbidity terms clearly begs many questions. While it would doubtless be claimed that the absence of data preclude more sophisticated weightings, against this it may again be said that absence or imperfection of *data* are no reasons for failing to make an explicit value judgment about the relative importance of mortality and morbidity.

Finally, it assumes that all years of life lost are equal value regardless of whose life is involved and regardless of any discounting for the futurity of many of these life-years.

Chen (1973) made a number of changes to the formula in order to measure the differential ill-health between a target and a reference population, eliminating D, introducing *relative* mortality and allowing for the fact that life expectancy in the absence of a specific disease is not likely to be the same for Indians and WASPS. His 'G index' was:

$$G = (M_i M_a)(D_1 + D_2)$$

where M_i and M_a are as before, but unadjusted for age and sex, D_1 is the difference between observed and 'expected' years lost from disease-specific mortality in Indian population, and D_2 is the difference between observed and 'expected' years lost from disease-specific morbidity in Indian population. The 'expected' values were those which would obtain if the disease impact on Indian and US populations were the same.

Although the Chen G index has a different purpose from the Q index, the value assumptions it makes are, in fact, the same: the morbidity measures making up D_2 are weighted in the same 1:3 ratio and the mortality and morbidity elements are assigned equal weights of unity in terms of time. The G index measures the potential increase in health status from the complete elimination of a disease while the Q index measures the increase if the target population is improved to the level of the reference population.

An alternative and perhaps more sympathetic interpretation would be to suppose that these weights are to be regarded as essentially *provisional*, to be altered in the light of professional (etc.) judgments about the validity of the index and after the experience of practical use. Indeed, both Miller and Chen argue strongly, and surely wisely, that such an index should not be used in isolation from or regardless of professional judgments. One might add that the judgments (of value) of politicians and patients who are important non-professionals should probably also have some role. As we shall see, other investigators have been far less cautious about the explicit use of normative weights in index construction and have gone to quite sophisticated lengths to derive these.

It is also finally worth noting that both the Q and G indexes are not independent of inputs: an increase in hospital provision to the Indian relative to non-Indian population would increase both indexes suggesting that 'need' has increased along with the means of meeting it. This, as we have observed before, is a highly undesirable feature of health indexes and is a basic fault which is mostly avoided in the indexes to be discussed in the remainder of this chapter.

There has of course been some debate as to whether it is really necessary to combine the dimensions into a single index – or at least into a set of indexes that is smaller than the total number of dimensions. In a very early study, for example, Stouman and Falk (1936) argued that a single combined index 'could have only a slight interest and might serve as much to obscure as to measure individuality of ... problems.' While this point is well taken, there are clearly many occasions when it is desired to classify groups, regions and individuals according to their over-all health status, to record changes in it to time and to relate changes in it to the various factors thought to influence it.

As we shall see, some thorny issues are raised once it is decided to combine different dimensions of ill health to make a single index and, ultimately, there is no escaping the fact that at some stage in the decision-making hierarchy *someone* will have to apply *some* weights if any decision is to be reached: for example, someone will have to decide whether, in regional patterns of resource distribution, a region with high morbidity but lower mortality rates should receive more or less priority than one with high mortality but lower morbidity.

This problem cannot be escaped by disaggregation. For example, even though disaggregating mortality and morbidity according to the diseases associated with them will indicate the specific kind of resources required to combat them but, so long as resources are not unlimited, it will not obviate the necessity of deciding which diseases are the more 'serious.' Precisely such an exercise, in which weights are assigned to diseases (but the weights are not variable with respect to prevalence or incidence) has been conducted for Ontario by Wolfson (1974), as we shall see below. In cases, however, where a rather eclectic set of indicators is used to form merely impressionistic judgments of need, it would seem preferable not to combine them. Such applies, for example, when one uses existing data to make comparisons. There is no obviously uniquely right way of adding up, say, crude mortality, perinatal mortality and maternal mortality rates in an international comparison study because the weights applicable in any one country, no matter how carefully they have been derived, may be quite inappropriate for another. This is merely one aspect of the familiar problem of interregional comparisons of standards of living.

When we come to look at the indicators for Ontario counties in chapter seven we shall similarly draw back from combining them into a single indicator – not least because some of them are *already* the result of a weighting procedure and what effectively we have is a set of *alternative* indicators of the health levels of counties.

There are two basic approaches to the question of weights once it has been decided that the dimensions measured *are* to be thoughtfully combined. One, which we term the 'functional/dysfunctional' approach, ranks the dimensions by priority; for example: incontinence is a worse handicap than inability to work which is, in term, worse than being unable to go out shopping. The second, which we term the 'economic' approach, is more flexible, allowing (*a*) that the degree of relative 'badness' of the above handicaps depends partly on their severity, and (*b*) that they may interact in such a way that a combination of disabilities may be worse (or better) than the sum of their 'badness' considered separately. The terms 'functional/dysfunctional' and 'economic' are used because the two approaches seem to be much in the spirit of the functionalist sociological and anthropological literature on the one hand and the economic theory of individual action on the other. Paradoxically, however, the functional/dysfunctional approach has been widely used by economists, medical researchers and OR researchers (as we have already seen in the Guttman scale), while sociologists have often been closer in their approach to the potential sensitivity of what we here describe as the 'economic' approach.

At least some economists have frowned on the first of these approaches (e.g., Olson, 1970; Culyer, 1973) partly because it can lead easily to logical error and triviality, and partly, which is more relevant in the present context, because it consists of a highly unrealistic way of describing the kinds of values that people actually have: for example, it implies a 'lexicographic' preference ordering of the type that says *all* disability of the 'worst' category should be ameliorated before any of another category. Actually, it seems far more plausible to suppose that the ranking of categories of disability varies continuously according to the severity of disabilities in those categories.

In terms of a figure introduced in the previous chapter, the difference between the two approaches can be illustrated as follows. The functionalist approach implies that all leftward movements from A to G in Figure 8 are

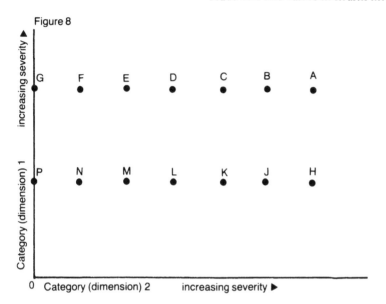

Figure 8

improvements and that all leftward movements from *H* to *P* are even better improvements but, if category 2 is regarded as the more 'serious' dimension of handicap, any leftward movement will be preferable to any downward movement. For example, $F \rightarrow G$ is preferable to $F \rightarrow N$, $A \rightarrow B$ preferable to $A \rightarrow H$. The economic approach allows, however, for the possibility that at some scores in dimension 2, reductions of handicap in dimension 1 way be preferable. For example, $A \rightarrow B$ may be preferable to $A \rightarrow H$, but $F \rightarrow N$ preferable to $F \rightarrow G$.

If, then, a lexicographic approach seems too crude, at least at the level of abstraction needed for defining the *general* characteristics a procedure for measuring health status ought to have, we must look more closely at the kind of 'measurement' that is implied by what we have called the 'economic' approach to contrast it with the 'functional-dysfunctional' approach. Basically we shall be concerned with *ordinal* and *cardinal* measurement.

A purely *ordinal* scale of measurement gives only the rank order of entities. Once a number has been assigned to any one entity, the only constraint on the numbers assigned to the others is that successively higher entities have successively higher numbers and successively lower entities have successively lower ones. We are also concerned with two kinds of *cardinal* measurement. Measurement on an interval scale implies that numbers assigned to entities are arbitrary save that they not only order them (as in ordinal measurement) but also keep the ratio of the intervals between them the same. This kind of measure is akin to that which we use for measuring temperature: a temperature of 212°F may appear 'twice as hot' as 106°F, yet if we compared the same degrees of hotness on a Celsius scale, we could scarcely claim that 100°C were 'twice as hot' as 41.1°C. With interval scales, like measures of temperature, there is no special significance attached to zero, for the origin is arbitrary. But we can compare *differences* between temperature consistently. Thus the difference between 212°F and 106°F is twice that between 106°F and 53°F. Similarly the difference between 100°C and 41.1°C is twice that between 41.1°C and 11.7°C. With a ratio scale, the origin is not arbitrary: for example, zero means 'none,' and only the unit is arbitrary, so we can speak of 'twice as much' here as there, etc., as in measures of weight and measures of mortality, disease incidence, etc. This latter is the 'strongest' form of measurement we shall encounter.

Typically, in economics, dimensions on axes are measured on a ratio scale (guns or butter) while value (utility) is measured either ordinally or on an interval scale. With health indexes, the axes may be ordinal (degrees of disability) or on a ratio scale (morbidity rates) while the values taken by the index combining the entities on the axes are typically on an interval scale.

The ways in which over-all scores are assigned in various combinations of scores of the several dimensions that may be used are crucially determined by the kind of measurement being used. This we shall see as we examine the studies that have been undertaken. The nature of the measurement must also be borne in mind when interpreting the results, and here even the sophisticated have, as we shall see, been led astray.

One important and exceedingly thorough British study (Harris *et al.*, 1971) sought to measure degrees of physical, mental, and sensory handicap in the population in order to assess its effect on ability to obtain work, need for health and welfare support and so on. This study classified severity of handicap into eight categories varying from (1) 'people needing help going to or using the WC practically every night ... need to be fed and dressed, or if they can feed and/or dress themselves, they need a lot of help during the day with washing and WC, or are incontinent' to (8) 'people to whom impairment presents no difficulty in taking care of themselves.' The first three of these categories, relating to those who need 'special care' were defined in terms of the presence or otherwise of specific inabilities or restrictions. The rest, however, were defined in terms of the ratio scale scoring system for the degree of impairment or disability in specified dimensions subsequently combined to make only *ordinal* judgments, and this is therefore of more interest in the present context. The dimensions, the units of measurement (verbal descriptions), and scores were as in Table 5.

The procedure then was to add up the predetermined scores according to the technical assignment of individuals within the cells of Table 5. The crucial value judgments relate, of course, (*a*) to the selection of the eight dimensions, and (*b*)

TABLE 5

Dimensions, units of measurement, and scores of the Harris index

| | Units of measurement of severity | | |
Dimensions	Can do with no difficulty (a)	Some difficulty but can do on own (b)	Cannot do on own even with difficulty (c)
1. Getting in/out of bed	0	2	3
2. Getting to/using WC	0	4	6
3a. Having bath	0	2	3
3b. Washing hand and face	0	2	3
4. Putting on shoes/stockings	0	2	3
5. Doing up zips/ buttons	0	4	6
6. Dressing (other than 4 and 5)	0	2	3
7. Feeding	0	4	6
8. Combing or shaving	0	2	3

SOURCE: Harris et al. (1971, Appendix D)

the relative (and fixed) weights assigned them. In fact, in this study, degree of severity was not assessed by experts such as social workers but by the *informants* themselves: the 'experts' provided the description of the units of measurement and the corresponding scores, respondents decided which cells they belonged to. According to the total score thus computed, the remaining 5 categories of handicap were defined as in Table 6.

Some examples of the kind of person allocated to each category are as follows (Harris et al., 1971, 15-16):

Category 4

A household woman, aged 74, suffering from hemiplegia, who cannot use her right hand at all. Lives with her married daughter, son-in-law and grandson. Is housebound, has a wheelchair, and can make limited progress around the house with the use of a walking frame. Daughter has to wash and dress her, and cut up her food, which she can then eat with spoon or fork, using her left hand.

TABLE 6

Scores needed for each category in Harris index

Score	Category
18–26	4
12–17	5
6–11	6
1–5	7
0	8

SOURCE: Harris *et al.* (1971, Appendix D)

A blind widow of 86, living with her widowed daughter, who is herself 60 years old. She is unsteady on her feet, and never goes out, although she manages to get about the house. She can wash her own hands and face and manage most other items of self-care with some difficulty, but her daughter has to help her to dress herself, do up buttons, etc., and give her a body-wash.

Category 5

A woman of 49, separated from her husband, living with her three unmarried children, aged between 14 and 23. Has polio, which has paralyzed her right side. Can manage to take care of herself on own, but has difficulty getting in and out of bed, using the WC, having an all-over wash, and dressing. Does own cooking and housework with difficulty and daughter takes her out shopping.

Married man of 46, who has blackouts and limited use of right side of body due to brain damage. Cannot do up buttons and zips, and has difficulty washing, dressing and shaving, but can manage on own. He has had to give up work.

Married man of 58, right hand affected by a stroke. Has to be helped with putting on shoes and socks, and having a bath, and finds dressing, shaving, etc., difficult. He can feed himself and use the WC without difficulty, and is working full-time as a cost clerk.

Category 6

A married man of 64 with rheumatoid arthritis. Has difficulty getting in and out of bed, using WC, and bathing, but manages on own. Otherwise he has no difficulty except with putting on shoes and socks which he has to have done for him. He gets around in his wheelchair and is able to get in and out of his chair without help. He retired from work aged 63.

A woman aged 41 with arthritis, who can only go out with difficulty. Cannot bath or give herself an all-over wash, dress herself, or comb her hair. Cannot do housework because of disability.

Category 7
Married woman of 58 with angina. Has difficulty bending and stretching to put on shoes, and dressing. Otherwise has no difficulty in taking care of herself or getting out and about. Does most of her own cooking, shopping and housework, but has difficulty lifting and pushing.

Married man of 48, torn ligaments and broken cartilage in left leg. Has difficulty walking and getting into bed.

Married man of 71, suffering from hardened arteries and obesity. Has difficulty putting on shoes and socks, and washing below the belt.

It was also possible to relate severity of handicap according to the medical condition to which it was principally attributed. These results are displayed in Table 7.

While the foregoing can give but the merest hint of the wealth of detail in the Harris project, there is much to be gained from even greater analytical simplification in order to identify the value-issues or trade-offs embodied in the procedure used.

Figure 9 is a matrix derived from considering just two dimensions (1 and 2). From this figure we see that individuals may, on these two dimensions alone, fall into eight categories with those who are least impaired receiving the index 0 and those most severely impaired receiving an index of 9. The interpretation of these numbers is *ordinal* — a score of 6 implying that a person is more handicapped that he would be with a score of 2, but not cardinal, *viz.* it is not intended to convey that he is three times worse off. The combination (b,b) is, however, regarded as equally handicapping as the combination (a,c) (assuming, of course, no difference in any other dimensions not shown in the figure).

If combinations such as (b,b) (where the first letter refers to ordinate) are to remain 'equal to' combinations such as (a,c), it follows that, as we have pointed out above, the ordering of degrees of severity in each dimension has to be a ratio scale *and* that the ratio of increments in one dimension to these in any other remain constant. Thus, we could not merely double all the numbers assigned to severity of difficulty in using the WC (0,4,6) and leave unchanged the numbers assigned to severity of difficulty in getting out of bed. If we did (as the reader may readily compute for himself) combinations (b,b) and (a,c) would no longer be equivalent. If we double one lot we must therefore double the others. Nor could we take the order (0,4,5) as equivalent to (0,4,6) in the WC severity dimension, as we could if they were merely ordinal numbers, without having to change the numbers in the other dimension: in particular, to preserve the equality of (b,b) and (a,c), $b = 2$ will have to become $b = 1$, while to keep $(c,b) < (b,c)$, $c < 2$ is required.

TABLE 7

Main causes of handicap by severity of handicap and disease classification

Main cause of impairment	Category of handicap								No. on which % based
	Handicapped					Minor/no handicap			
	1-3	4	5	6	1-6	7	8a non-motor	8b motor	
Infective and parasitic diseases	0.8	1.8	5.9	17.6	26.1	27.6	38.7	7.6	123
Neoplasms	10.5	2.6	18.5	9.6	41.2	19.3	37.7	1.8	114
Allergic, endocrine, metabolic and nutritional diseases	4.7	–	4.7	17.4	26.8	19.2	52.6	1.4	213
Diseases of blood and blood-forming organs	1.7	0.9	14.8	32.2	49.6	12.2	33.9	4.3	115
Mental, psycho-neurotic, and personality disorders	6.2	1.8	5.8	16.2	30.0	14.9	51.6	3.5	407
Diseases of central nervous system									
Poliomyelitis	3.8	–	6.0	12.7	22.5	30.7	–	46.8	156
Cerebral haemorrhage, strokes	29.0	9.5	13.4	18.9	70.8	12.9	–	16.3	541
Multiple sclerosis	32.6	10.2	22.5	13.3	78.6	12.2	–	9.2	98
Paralysis agitans (Parkinsonism)	22.0	9.9	19.8	18.6	70.3	19.8	–	9.9	91
Cerebral palsy (spastic)	15.9	3.2	4.8	20.6	44.5	22.2	–	33.3	64
Paraplegia, hemiplegia	12.5	7.0	14.0	22.2	55.7	16.3	–	28.0	88
Epilepsy	2.3	6.6	1.3	7.9	18.1	10.6	68.7	2.6	88
Migraine	–	–	–	[6]	[6]	[2]	[6]	–	14
Dizziness, convulsions, vertigo	4.2	–	12.2	18.2	34.6	16.7	48.7	–	71
Sciatica	–	–	2.1	6.4	8.5	46.8	–	44.7	60
Head injury	[4]	[2]	–	[4]	[10]	[2]	[35]	[1]	48
Other central nervous system diseases	9.1	6.1	13.3	12.7	41.2	15.2	–	43.6	176
Diseases of circulatory system									
Coronary disease	1.3	2.0	6.0	13.0	22.3	29.2	48.2	0.3	535
Arterio-sclerotic diseases	4.6	0.9	2.8	18.4	26.7	30.4	41.5	1.4	219

Hypertension	3.4	5.7	4.4	18.0	31.5	24.6	41.3	2.6	235
Diseases of arteries	0.9	4.0	4.0	8.9	17.8	41.6	33.7	6.9	108
Varicose veins	—	0.9	12.2	6.6	19.7	17.0	53.8	9.5	109
Heart trouble (unspecified)	5.4	3.8	4.2	11.9	25.3	25.0	47.8	1.9	365
Other diseases of circulatory system	4.5	0.2	9.0	22.8	36.5	25.6	35.7	2.2	468
Diseases of respiratory system	1.5	1.4	5.2	13.9	22.0	20.3	56.6	1.1	1175
Diseases of digestive system	3.3	2.5	6.0	19.3	31.1	29.9	38.4	0.6	340
Diseases of genito-urinary system	9.0	–	12.8	27.0	48.8	23.5	27.0	0.7	144
Diseases of sense organs (excluding blindness)	0.9	1.5	5.0	18.0	25.4	17.3	56.0	1.3	851
Diseases of skin and cellular tissue	2.4	–	3.7	8.6	14.7	23.5	54.4	7.4	84
Diseases of bones and organs of movement									
Arthritis	4.0	4.7	11.1	28.0	47.8	23.5	—	28.7	3610
Osteomyelitis	–	–	–	[6]	[6]	[4]	—	[9]	19
Slipped disc, lumbago	0.4	2.7	8.6	20.3	32.0	27.0	—	41.0	271
Muscular dystrophy	[5]	–	[2]	[11]	[18]	[4]	—	[10]	32
Fractures	5.7	4.7	7.4	24.9	42.7	21.5	—	35.8	380
Sprains, strains, dislocations, etc.	–	1.6	9.7	13.8	25.1	25.2	—	49.7	133
Other diseases of bones and organs of movement	3.4	0.6	8.0	23.2	35.2	26.2	—	38.6	476

TABLE 7, *continued*

Main causes of handicap and disease classification

Main cause of impairment	Category of handicap								Minor/no handicap				No. on which % based
	Handicapped												
	1-3	4	5	6	1-6		7	8a non-motor	8b motor			
Congenital malformations	3.0	3.0	1.5	19.7	27.2		25.8	–	47.0			66
Injuries	0.6	1.3	5.1	13.1	20.1		19.7	32.3	27.9			626
Senility and ill-defined conditions	14.1	5.7	7.7	10.6	38.1		27.6	30.0	4.3			506
Amputations	1.9	–	4.7	16.9	23.5		18.5	–	58.0			533
Blindness	5.4	3.2	6.4	11.5	26.5		18.8	54.7	–			298

[ ] denotes number not percentage
SOURCE: Harris *et al.* (1971) Table AVI

NOTE: (8) is divided into (a) and (b) with (a) referring to disorders other than musculo-skeletal and neurological and (b) referring to the latter. Epilepsy, migraine, dizziness, convulsions, and vertigo were included in (a). Broadly the idea is to distinguish (a) non-motor handicaps, and (b) motor handicaps. While persons in category 8 have no difficulty with physical self-care, they may, of course, suffer considerably from other ill-health and other physical restrictions.

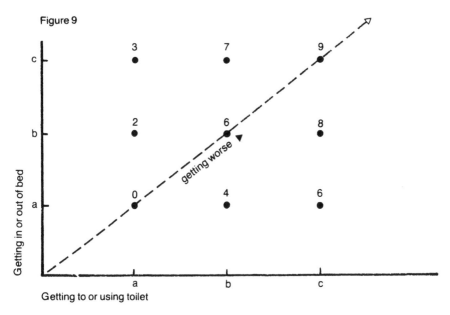

Figure 9

None of these implications were, of course, identified in the Harris study and we should note that the apparent restrictiveness of an implicit ratio scale interpretation of the axes and of their proportionality one to another is much reduced by the merely ordinal *interpretation* of the resultant index of handicap. In general, however, it would seem undesirable to suppose that an index can be derived by simply adding up the scores on dimensions. In particular, if the total is no more than the sum of the parts, no allowance is made for the possibility that one may wish to regard a *combination* of disability as worse than the sum of each considered separately.

The way in which the index was used (i.e., to classify people into groups, having only an ordinal relationship one group with another) and its purposes (which did not include attempts to measure the effects of care on changing disability states or attempts to evaluate the 'worthwhileness' of such efforts) substantially reduce the significance of these criticisms, however, and it would plainly be unjust to criticize this study for lacking a sophistication it did not require. The study does serve, however, to bring out the richness – but also the practical complexity – of even a rather elementary method. Within this method, the Harris study displays highly commendable thoroughness and common sense.

The objective of the Harris study was principally to identify groups of disabled persons in the population who were in need of support. About the same time in England, a doctor and an anaesthetist produced a more ambitious proposal (Grogono and Woodgate, 1971). The objective of their study was put as follows: 'we have as yet no national basis upon which to organize and distribute our resources. This must in part be attributed to the absence of any method of measuring efficacy: we have no method of measuring a patient's health before and after treatment.'

Grogono and Woodgate identified (after discussion with patients and colleagues) ten dimensions of human functioning which they felt gave a comprehensive view of the aspects of life upon which medicine may be expected to have impact. In particular, they felt these provided a foundation for more specific descriptions of patient states than the customary 'fit for light duty only' or 'better than yesterday' which, they claim, are characteristic descriptions used by medical practitioners. The dimensions are set out in Table 8.

In each dimension, impairment was measured on a three-point ratio scale with normal = 1, impaired = ½ and incapacitated = 0. For each patient the score at a point in time was the simple arithmetic sum of the scores across all ten dimensions. By implication, each of the ten factors was given an equal weight (for failure to ascribe *any* weights is equivalent to ascribing *equal* weights) and the degree of seriousness of malfunction is both linear and simply additive (a person with five 'ones' on the first five dimensions and five 'zeros' on the second five is judged just as bad as a person having five 'zeros' on the first five dimensions and 'ones' on the rest, and just as bad as one scoring ½ across the board).

In terms of our two-dimensional Figure 10, the trade-offs between dimensions are (*a*) constant, (*b*) on a one-for-one basis. The contours connecting points regarded as equally bad (or good) are straight lines at 45° (and have equal incremental values since the index score attached to each contour is simply the sum of the coordinates). Thus, in Figure 10, points *A* and *B* are equally good and are half as much again better than either *C*, *D*, or *E* (all of which are equally bad). In turn, *C*, *D*, and *E* are each twice as good as *F* or *G*.

Although in testing this procedure, they found that it was easy to assign the scores and that a high degree of consensus was found among those doing this, and despite the fact that 'there did not seem to be any anomalies' the exercise does throw into high relief three crucial value judgments, pictorially displayed in Figure 10. These are: (*a*) the judgment that the 'rate of substitution' of one dimension for another is constant (the index contours in Figure 10 are straight lines): *viz.* a half unit increase in one dimension can always be exactly offset by a *given* decrease in *any* other dimension; (*b*) the judgment that the index contours are set at 45°, that an increase in one dimension is always exactly offset by *an identical* decrease in any other dimension; (*c*) the judgment that a move from one index contour to another gives *equal* increments of health status.

The Grogono-Woodgate paper has no awareness that these value judgments are built into its procedure. Once they are exposed, however, it seems by no

TABLE 8

Components of the Grogono-Woodgate index

	normal = 1	impaired = 1/2	incapacitated = 0
1 Ability to work			
2 Hobbies and recreation			
3 Malaise, pain, or suffering			
4 Worry or unhappiness			
5 Ability to communicate			
6 Ability to sleep			
7 Independence of others			
8 Ability to eat/enjoy food			
9 Bladder and bowels			
10 Sex life			
TOTAL			

Figure 10
Implicit tradeoffs in the Grogono-Woodgate Index (2 dimensions only)

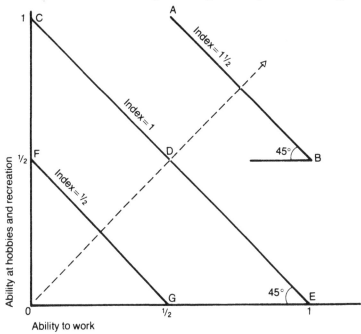

means likely that these would be the value judgments even the authors would have wished to make had they been confronted with the necessity of doing so.

At the general level, what would appear to be the most reasonable presumptions to make about these three value judgments? Without defining what the judgments should precisely be, the following *characteristics* of the value judgments would appear to be reasonable.

(*a*) The 'rate of substitution' between dimensions will not normally be constant. It might *diminish* as increasing disability in one dimension is recorded. Intuitively, this implies that earlier 'units' of disability are regarded as more serious than 'equal' additions to higher disability levels. But the reverse may be true: loss of a second eye is worse than loss of a first eye. In this case, it seems that the units (eyes lost) are not equal-interval measures of disability. Let us illustrate for a supposed diminishing rate of substitution. The object is not to assert that this will invariably be so, only that *constancy* seems an implausible general assumption. The case is shown in Figure 11 (where the axes now measure disabilities). Suppose that A and B were regarded as positions of equal over-all disability (i.e. would receive the same index number describing state of health), and suppose that C and D were likewise regarded as equal levels of disability. A diminishing rate of substitution suggests that the ratio AE/EB would be smaller than the ratio CF/FD.

This characteristic corresponds to one version of the economist's conception of the diminishing rate of substitution between goods.[2] Note that, as we have put it, this property is *not* dependent upon the dimensions being measured on a ratio scale. The degrees of disability on the axes may be measured on an interval scale, and still, with equal scores in the other dimension(s), the 'degree of seriousness' attached to incremental disability in the remaining dimension will fall: if B is regarded as worse than E by the same amount that D is worse than F, then, if D and C are judged equally bad, B will be judged *better than G*. Again, since the individual is worse off at B than at D a lesser increase in the other dimension will 'compensate' for a given improvement in his condition.

(*b*) Implied by characteristic (*a*) when the dimensions are measured on a scale that is unique up to an interval or ratio scale is that the rate at which dimensions are substituted, along any contour line connecting points having an equal index score, will also diminish. Thus, the contours will not be linear as in the Grogono-Woodgate index, but generally concave from above as in Figure 12 (*viz.*, getting flatter as one moves horizontally to the east and steeper as one moves vertically to the north).

---

2 It is, in fact, somewhat more restrictive than the usual assumption, corresponding here to characteristic (*b*) which does not imply (*a*), though (*a*) implies (*b*).

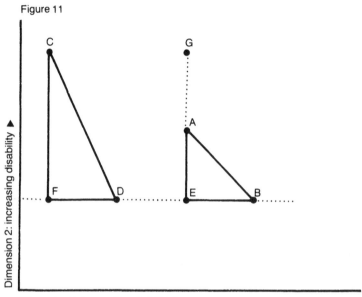

Figure 11

Dimension 2: increasing disability ▲

Dimension 1: increasing disability ▶

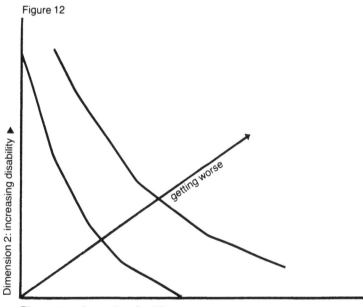

Figure 12

Dimension 2: increasing disability ▲

getting worse

Dimension 1: increasing disability ▶

(c) Apart from a general presumption that the index should increase as one moves north, east, or north-east (whether it measures increasing health or increasing ill-health) there is no general presumption about how the increments change — whether, for example, they become smaller, larger, stay the same, or are variable.

It should be emphasized that characteristic (b) is relevant only where the dimensions of disability (viz., the axes) are measured in equal intervals. There is, for example, no presumption of concavity (nor of linearity either we should add!) for axes with only ordinal measures of dysfunction measured along them (hence the convex instances in Culyer, Lavers, and Williams, 1972, are not to be seen as contrary to the characteristics suggested here as desirable) and economists should not be put off by the possibility of 'convex indifference curves.'

The third characteristic of indexes is left deliberately flexible in order not to prejudge the issue of how increases in several dimensions at the same time affect the index. Certainly it should increase in value (indicating worse health if the dimensions are 'bad' or better health if they are 'good') but whether it will increase at a constant, increasing, or decreasing constant rate for equal increases in the dimensions will depend, we may plausibly suppose, on the nature of the dimensions we are considering. (Clearly to speak of it increasing at a particular rate requires it to be measured at least on an interval scale.)

For example, suppose that the two dimensions are 'ability to see' and 'mobility' and we measure improvements in these functions along the axes. It then seems reasonable to expect the increase in the index to be greater for a given increase in both dimensions than the sum of the same increase in each considered separately because each improvement enhances the enjoyment of the other.[3] Alternatively, if the dimensions do not impinge on one another at all, we may expect given successive increases in each dimension to produce equal successive increases in the index. The third case is, of course, when the increases in the index become smaller. Such may occur, for example, when the dimensions are, say, 'reduction of maternal mortality rate' and 'reduction of infant mortality rate' where the benefit from both together is possibly less than the sum of each one's separate benefit (in the sense that as over-all mortality rates fall, the whole question of premature death becomes less of a priority).

This issue, aside from its general importance, has acquired specific relevance in the context of the kind of index developed by Bush and his colleagues. For many of the purposes to which health indexes and indicators may be put, it is

---

3 In the days of cardinal utility in economics, this amounted to a definition of 'complementarity' (see Georgescu-Roegen, 1952).

necessary that the index be constructed on an interval scale; that is, that it should be possible to make statements like: this increase in the index is the same/greater/smaller than this other increase; or on a ratio scale enabling statements like: this value of the index is twice as high as this other value. This desirable property does not, however, imply that characteristic (c) be violated as seems to be implied by Patrick, Bush and Chen (1973, 242). Here, as a test of the interval nature of the index they derive, they suggest that the difference in index score between two pairwise comparisons of disability which are different in all respects save one, where they differ by the same degree, should be zero.

Their precise example is as follows. Compare individual 1 who travels with difficulty but can move independently in a wheelchair and can perform self-care activities but who has pain in his back or hips, with individual 2 who also has pain in his back or hips but who is hospitalized, walks with difficulty and needs help with self care. Now compare individual 3 who is like individual 1 save that he has a foot or leg impairment, with individual 4 who is like the individual 2 save that he too has foot or leg impairment. The difference in the index between 1 and 2 should be the same as that between 3 and 4 according to these researchers. But why should this be so? Surely there is no implausibility or irrationality in supposing that mobility restrictions for those with pain in the sites described may be considered differently in terms of seriousness from such restrictions upon those with foot or leg impairments. Patrick et al. do explicitly assume 'no interaction' between the dimensions of disability. But that is precisely what is denied by characteristic (c). Why should we want to rule this out? The test proposed for the interval nature of the scale is not really a test of this at all. Instead it is a test for independent additivity of the 'utilities' of various degrees of disability. Sometimes the utility of the whole may be the sum of the utility of the parts, but in general we have no reason at all to suppose that people's attitudes to disability are of this kind.

While it may seem 'obvious' that a health index is constructed on at least an interval scale, in practical experiments there are good reasons for supposing that this is not the case. One reason why not arises because those assigning numbers to characteristics and combinations of characteristics tend, when constrained to keep within limits (say, 0 and 1 or 0 and 100) to avoid extreme values and there is a bunching towards the centre of the distribution brought about by this psychological quirk. A well-known example (at least in Britain) is the reluctance of markers of undergraduates' examination papers to award marks in excess of the low seventies (in Britain, such marks usually indicate a first-class honours paper) even though the scale extends in principle up to 100. Hence the 'real' difference between 65 and 75 may be much larger than the difference between 55 and 65. Fortunately, there are statistical techniques for 'stretching' the scales in appropriate ways (Blishke, Bush, and Kaplan, 1975).

In experimental work, five methods have been used to assign index numbers to health states. These are as follows: (*a*) the 'category' method; (*b*) the 'magnitude' method; (*c*) the 'equivalence' method; (*d*) the 'standard gamble' method; (*e*) the 'time trade-off' method.

The first three of these have been used by Bush and his colleagues and we shall draw on their work in describing the procedures and their results. The other two have been used by several authors including Wolfson and Torrance in Ontario, for that, we shall draw on their work.[4]

The 'category' method
According to this method, individuals are given case-descriptions (corresponding to the verbal statements on the axes of Figures 8-12) and asked to ascribe numbers within a stated range such that equal differences in the numbers correspond to equal improvements or deteriorations in the over-all health status ascribed to the subjects. Patrick, Bush, and Chen (1973) used both graduate students in public administration and public health and professional members of the New York State Health Planning Commission and Advisory Council. The precise instructions given were:

Evaluate the desirability of each day by circling a number from 1 to 11 which shows how desirable each day seem to you. Each number represents an equal step on a scale of desirability such that 5 is one step more desirable than 4, 11 is one step more desirable than 10, and so forth. The label 'most desirable' is above category 11 and represents a day in the life a person who was as healthy as possible on that day, i.e., performed his major and other activities, had no discernible symptoms, and walked and traveled about freely. The label 'least desirable' is below category 1 and represents a person who died during the day. All items fall between these two extremes, and you may use all 11 categories as you see fit. (Patrick *et al.*, 1973, 253)

They were not constrained to use integers but a feature of this method is that those assigning the numbers have to bear in mind that the same 'distance' between any two pairs of numbers on the index must represent the same improvement or deterioration in health status as judged by the assigners.

The 'magnitude' method
According to this method, the assigners are given case-descriptions as before and asked to ascribe numbers within a stated range such that the ratio of any two

---

4 For a short review of the historical development of the first two of these and their application in an entirely different area see Sellin and Wolfgang (1964).

numbers corresponds to the ratio of health states that the numbers measure. The instructions given by Patrick *et al.* in this case were as follows:

Evaluate the desirability of each day by writing in the score box a number which reflects how preferable each day seems to you. This standard item describes a day which has been given a score of 1000. It is a day in the life of a person who was as healthy as possible on that day. Every other day should be scored in relation to this standard description. For example, if the item seems half as desirable as the standard, then write in a score of 500. If the day appears a tenth as preferable as the standard, then write in a score of 100. You may use any whole number or fraction that is greater than zero and equal to or less than 1000. (Patrick *et al.*, 1973, 235)

By anchoring the magnitude scale at each end, clearly this method, as used by Patrick *et al.*, is conceptually equivalent to the category method differing only in its experimental features and thus providing a test for the reliability of the category method. The conceptual equivalence of the two methods can be readily seen: if 4 is twice as good as 2 which is twice as good as 1; then the difference between 4 and 2 must be twice the difference between 2 and 1, so that each unit measures an equal 'amount' of good health. [5]

Torrance (1970, 99) proposed a 'direct measurement' technique in which the judge was asked first to rank all the described states including 'healthy' and 'dead.' He was then asked how many times worse he considered each relative to the one immediately higher in the preference ordering. States 'healthy' and 'dead' were given the values 1 and 0 respectively and the times worse figures were used to compute the values from the other states. Because the high abstraction involved with this method for the general practitioners used as his judges, however, the actual procedures used were the 'time trade-off' and 'standard gamble' approaches (see below).

The 'equivalence' method
According to this method, the assigners were given the same cases descriptions as before and asked to assume that a unit of health is the same regardless of the person whom it describes. Subjects were then asked how many sick persons are equivalent in total health status to a given number of perfectly healthy persons. The precise instructions given by Patrick *et al.* were:

5 A similar procedure has been used by Gustafson and Holloway (1975) to estimate
the severity of burns: the severity of each dimension of a burn (e.g., site, thickness, area) was first scaled in this way and the dimensions then weighted and summed to yield the index. A study using a 'true' magnitude method is Wyler *et al.* (1970).

Suppose there are two groups of people, both of which will die immediately if not helped. You have the resources to keep one and only one of these groups alive for one more year, after which they will also die. The first group contains 100 people in a state of maximum health (standard). I want you to make a decision concerning the number of people in the second group. Persons in the second group are in a state of health lower than the standard (items in the booklet). With each item in this booklet, ask yourself this question: 'How many people in this state of health do I consider equivalent to the 100 people of the same age in the standard group?' Start with 100 and increase this number to the point at which you are not able to decide between the standard and comparison groups. You may use any number equal to or greater than 100 (Patrick *et al.*, 1973, 236)

Letting I_h represent the index for a perfectly healthy person and I_s the index for a sick person, then with N_h representing the numbers of healthy persons and Ns the number of sick persons of a given type regarded as equivalent, the experiment asks the subjects to select N_s such that $I_h N_h = I_s N_s$. From this the ratios of the indexes can be readily obtained: $I_s/I_h = N_h/N_s$, and with one point on the scale fixed ($I_h = 1.0$) and N_h given ($= 100$), we have $I_h = 1.0$ so that

$$I_s = \frac{N_h}{N_s} = 100/N_s.$$

This method is quite different from the preceding ones and requires, in particular, that the value assigned to *additional* persons whose lives are prolonged is always constant. The consequences if this crucial assumption is not made are illustrated in Figure 13. In panel (*a*) we assume that the average (index) value attached to prolonging a person's life by one year falls as shown by AV (average value). In panel (*b*) the AV of sick persons also falls but is lower than for healthy persons. Letting $I_h = 1.0$ and $N_h = 100$ we locate point A in panel (*a*) and, having performed the experiment, we locate point B in panel (*b*) such that the total value in each panel (indicated by the cross-hatched areas) is the same. We see that according to this experiment sick persons of the type included in N_s are judged to be half as healthy as the perfectly healthy individuals. An entirely different picture emerges, however, if we now compare the value of *one individual alone* in each group: we have (in the example in the figure) 1.3 for the healthy individual and 0.83 for the sick individual, with the sick person reckoned to be 0.63 as well as the healthy person.

Now a *diminishing* marginal value for additional individuals 'saved' as shown by the MV curves in the figure, may be a plausible assumption to make, for, since

Figure 13

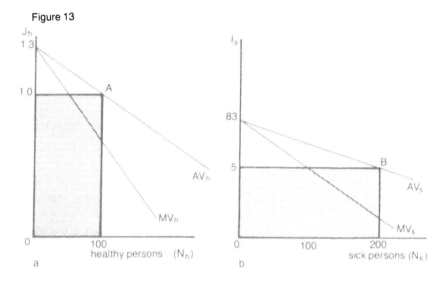

marginal values seem generally to fall everywhere else, so may the concern society feels for sick persons fall at the margin. If so, it violates an assumption that is central to the valid application of the equivalence method.[6]

These considerations serve usefully to remind us that all the methods of revealing values are not merely relative but also subject to *ceteris paribus* conditions, in particular, they are subject to assumptions concerning the number of persons in a category. If we interpret a health index as a *pseudo-quantity* measure of an individual's health rather than as a utility number, which seems to me the preferable interpretation of these figures then we may generally expect that, with aggregation over individuals in an evaluation exercise, the 'absolute value' of health (or its 'utility') or the value of *health status relative to other desired objects to which resources may be devoted* may not be constant at the margin. Only at this stage does it seem appropriate to introduce the notion of 'utility' explicitly, for it is at this stage that the highest-level trade-offs between health and other social policy objectives are made. At this level, the health index is itself measured on one axis of a multi dimensional trade-off program. The 'equivalence' method introduces elements of this trade-off at too early a stage in the analysis.

6 Essentially a similar difficulty arises with variants on this equivalence procedure such as 'equivalence through time' and 'equivalence in dysfunctional history' (see Fanshel and Bush, 1970; Fanshel 1972).

It is perhaps, worth pointing out that this objection to the 'equivalence' method in no way questions the assumption (though it *is* a value assumption!) that a day of bad health for *A* is neither better nor worse than a day of equally bad health for *B*. What it does suggest is that one may wish to deny that the *value* of improving both *A*'s and *B*'s health is twice the value of improving either *A*'s or *B*'s health; just as the value (to normal people) of seven steaks a week is not seven times the value of one steak a week. In *defining* 'health,' just as in *defining* 'steak' we will want to exclude the effect of the diminishing marginal valuation placed upon increasing amounts.

The 'standard gamble' method

This approach to deriving an index from descriptions of health states is based upon the utility theory sections of the classic by Von Neumann and Morgenstern (1953). It can be explained with the aid of Figure 14. In that figure, the points *A* and *B* are located and ranked. Here we assume that *B* is judged to indicate worse health than *A* in the simple two-dimension world there depicted, thus if we are to derive an index of *ill*-health, *B* will be assigned a higher number and is located on a higher index contour. The judges having valued *A* and *B*, we now assign arbitrary numbers to them. Letting $H(A)$ stand for the number assigned to *A* and $H(B)$ the number assigned to *B*, we have $H(B) > H(A)$. Let $H(A) = 1$ and $H(B) = 2$. Now locate some other combination *C* such than $H(C) > H(A)$ and $H(C) > H(B)$. The standard gamble approach offers a way of assigning a number to *C* such that all three combinations (*A*, *B* and *C*) can be located on a linear scale: whatever the initial numbers assigned to *A* and *B* (so long as $H(B) > H(A)$) the ratio of the difference between $H(C)$ and $H(B)$, and $H(B)$ and $H(A)$ will be the same.

The procedure is as follows: confront the judge with a choice between (i) a gamble between *C* and *A*, such that he will get *either* *C* or *A* with some probability (but not both), and (ii) the certainty of *B*. The judge is then asked what probability of getting *C* (or *A*) will make him indifferent between the gamble and the certainty. In effect, he is asked to choose a *p* such that:

$$H(B) = p \cdot H(A) + (1 - p) \cdot H(C).$$

Clearly, from this equation, given values for $H(B)$, $H(A)$, and *p*, $H(C)$ is determined:

$$H(C) = \frac{[H(B) - pH(A)]}{(1 - p).}$$

Figure 14

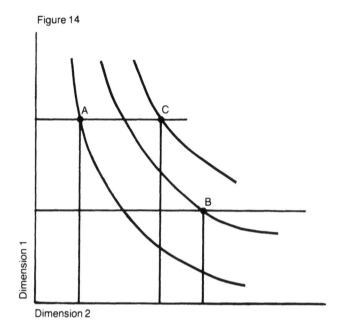

Dimension 1

Dimension 2

Suppose he becomes indifferent (the above equations hold) with $p = 0.6$. Then $H(C) = 3.5$. The judge, of course, need not be told any of the numbers initially assigned. He provides only the ordinal ranking and chooses the appropriate probability. To those who may doubt the uniqueness of this method of assigning numbers to health status (up to a linear transformation), Table 9 provides some calculations given arbitrary numbers for $H(A)$ and $H(B)$, the judge's view that A is better than B is better than C, and $p = 0.6$.

The procedure can be applied to as many health states as one wishes without the necessity of comparing each of them directly with one another.

This procedure was used by Wolfson (1974) to rank the seriousness of ill-health associated (by doctors) with a set of 59 disease categories. Each physician was presented with the following option: suppose he contracted a specified disease on the list, he had the choice of suffering it, with all its attendant consequences (including where relevant the possibility of death) and with its normal medical treatment, or of taking a hypothetical pill which would instantly remove the condition but had an attendant probability p of death. The probability was adjusted until indifference was obtained. Torrance (1970) and Torrance, Thomas, and Sackett (1972) have proposed and used essentially similar techniques (and, indeed, pioneered them in the health field) with

TABLE 9

The uniqueness of the standard gamble method of measurement

$H(A)$	$H(B)$	$H(C)$	$H(B)-H(A)$	$H(C)-H(B)$	$\dfrac{H(C)-H(B)}{H(B)-H(A)}$
1	2	3.5	1	1.5	1.5
1	4	8.5	3	4.5	1.5
3	6	10.5	3	4.5	1.5
6	100	241.0	94	141.0	1.5
100	101	102.5	1	1.5	1.5

imaginative variations in experimental design in order to facilitate the judge's ability to respond in as ready a fashion as possible.

Although the standard gamble technique does not permit making statements like 'this state is twice as ill as that,' (i.e., it does not provide a ratio scale), it does enable statements to be made about *changes* in health states of the sort: 'this change is twice as much as that change.' For most practical purposes, this is as much as is required (i.e. an interval scale).

The introduction of risk into the measurement procedure has both advantages and disadvantages. One advantage is that procedure permits a method of combining indexes of components of the characteristics bundle of 'health' into an over-all index: the expected 'utility' of two certain possibilities is simply their sum weighted by the probabilities of each component. This may prove to be of use in some applications. A possible disadvantage is that the health status index is itself not merely a function of the characteristics on the axes *but also of the judges' attitudes to risk:* a judge who was highly averse to risk, for example, would require a higher probability before he became indifferent between the sure thing and the gamble compared with a judge who enjoyed gambling. In situations where risk is inherent in the policy choice this is no disadvantage – indeed, it is an advantage. The standard gamble approach (though necessarily using physicians) is thus highly suited to epidemiological applications of health indexes, in prognosis and in 'production function' studies where the outcome is undertain. In descriptive studies, where the actual state of health is the focus rather than effecting some change in status, attitude to risk may distort the 'pure' trade-offs between dimensions of ill-health.[7]

This limitation of the standard gamble approach is inherent in Wolfson's study. Wolfson himself drew attention to the quite substantial coefficients of

7 A useful introduction to the underlying assumptions of the Neumann-Morgenstern standard gamble is Alchian (1953).

variation between probabilities selected by different judges (exceeding 50 per cent for 27 out of 59 disease categories) and, although he did not test to see whether some doctors were systematically more risk-averse than others, this (as well as the relatively small size of his sample) might have been a contributing factor to this large variability (see Table 10).

(We should emphasize, perhaps, that the attitude to risk in question is not a matter of professional judgment concerning probable incidence or probable recovery but the risk of death acceptable to the doctor in question in ensuring avoidance of disease). Whether their view of risk is the 'appropriate' one is discussed in the next section.

The 'time trade-off method'
Torrance (1970) pioneered this method, which is not unlike the 'equivalence' method. Here, the judges (physicians) were asked first to rank in order of preference a set of health states. Let the states, after ranking, be numbered $1, 2, ..., n$ in descending order of preference. The judges were then asked what length of time x in the healthy state would be equivalent to the longer length of time t in a dysfunctional state, assuming death would immediately follow in each case. Assigning an index of 1 ($h_1 = 1$) for the most preferred state and $h_n = 0$ for death the index for an intermediate state such as h_{n-1} could then be readily computed from the indifference equation $h_{n-1}t = h_1 x$. With $h_1 = 1$, it readily follows that $h_{n-1} = x/t$, and with a fixed t, the index for h_{n-1} is proportional to the amount of healthy time judged equivalent.[8]

The procedure estimates *average* utilities in terms of time and would, like the equivalence method, be distorted if, in the relevant time periods, additional sick-years had a substantially higher marginal disutility. Torrance found a high correlation between the results of this method and the standard gamble, each of which gave internally consistent results, and concluded that they were equivalent methods. Both methods revealed, however, a substantial variation between the scores assigned to specific condition/treatment combinations by the eleven judges as Wolfson found in his application of the standard gamble (see

---

8 Although this method could be used for all intermediate states, a modified method was actually used for those intermediate states other than $n - 1$, which avoided the continuous use of 'death' as a reference point. Judges were asked to consider what x would make them indifferent between state h_{i+1} for time $t < x$ and the better state h_i for time x, in each case followed by perfect health. The relevant equality is then

$$h_i x = h_{i+1} t + h_1 (x - t), \text{ giving}$$

$$h_i = 1 - (t/x)(1 - h_{i+1}).$$

TABLE 10

Risk weights and coefficients of variation of 59 disease states, from Wolfson (1974)

Disease state	Risk weight[1]	Coefficient[2] of variation (%)
1. Leukaemia	0.7700	10.38
2. Malignant neoplasm of the trachea	0.7241	20.18
3. Tetanus	0.6996	17.65
4. Muscular dystrophy	0.6352	21.12
5. Cirrhosis	0.5340	24.05
6. [3]Multiple sclerosis	0.4311	24.50
7. Malignant neoplasm of prostate	0.1820	6.11
8. [3]Chronic rheumatic heart disease	0.1647	25.33
9. Patent ductus arteriosus	0.1570	71.19
10. [3]Cerebral haemorrhage	0.1366	26.93
11. [3]Haemolytic disease of the newborn	0.1070	69.14
12. Polio	0.1013	40.82
13. Hydronephrosis	0.0946	46.21
14. Emphysema	0.0844	16.72
15. [3]Rheumatoid arthritis	0.0843	50.15
16. Septicaemia	0.0834	42.25
17. [3]Traumatic amputation of the arm	0.0714	29.00
18. Open wound of eye or ear	0.0705	52.76
19. Prematurity	0.0659	57.34
20. Hypertensive disease	0.0652	58.26
21. Haemorrhage of pregnancy	0.0541	68.92
22. Meningitis	0.0531	69.19
23. [3]Diabetes mellitus	0.0513	36.64
24. [3]Toxaemia of pregnancy	0.0457	41.92
25. Tuberculosis	0.0455	35.73
26. [3]Asthma	0.0363	32.41
27. Spina bifida	0.0322	59.26
28. [3]Peptic ulcer	0.0252	40.23
29. Malpresentation of the foetus	0.0184	57.17
30. Stricture of the urethra	0.0183	58.74
31. Displacement of intervetebral disc	0.0181	48.83
32. Epilepsy	0.0171	43.91
33. [3]Infectious hepatitis	0.0161	37.63
34. Club foot	0.0158	61.91
35. Fracture of the femur	0.0150	71.60
36. Osteoarthritis	0.0144	63.12
37. [3]Cleft palate	0.0091	46.48
38. Scarlet fever	0.0068	85.44
39. [3]Cystitis	0.0064	78.12
40. Uterovaginal prolapse	0.0064	60.00
41. Chronic sinusitis	0.0063	59.68

TABLE 10, *continued*

Risk weights and coefficients of variation of 59 disease states, from Wolfson (1974)

Disease state	Risk weight	Coefficient[2] of variation (%)
42. Hernia	0.0057	60.52
43. [3] Pneumonia	0.0055	37.27
44. Cataract	0.0045	50.45
45. Bursitis	0.0039	60.51
46. Migraine	0.0037	82.97
47. Varicose veins	0.0032	52.81
48. [3] Iron deficiency anaemia	0.0028	77.08
49. Cholelithiasis	0.0026	66.53
50. [3] Haemorrhoids	0.0024	42.91
51. Appendicitis	0.0024	72.08
52. Non-toxic goitre	0.0022	78.18
53. [3] Fracture of the jaw	0.0011	18.88
54. Benign neoplasma of the breast	0.0008	46.25
55. [3] Otitis media	0.0007	34.28
56. [3] Streptoccocal sore throat	0.0006	40.00
57. Pilonidal cyst	0.0005	28.00
58. Influenza	0.0005	28.00
59. [3] Impetigo	0.0001	14.00

NOTES: (1) Risk weight is the average risk of death accepted by the sample of doctors to rid themselves of the disease in question. (2) Coefficient of variation is the standard deviation times 100 divided by the mean. (3) Sample size equals 10, for all others equals 5.

Table 11). Torrance believed that the somewhat large confidence interval (at the 95 per cent level) would fall substantially for a larger sample than his eleven physicians.

In a subsequent experiment using larger samples of the public, Torrance (1976*b*) found that, as between his time trade-off method, the standard gamble method and category scaling, the time trade-off method has the highest degree of reliability, closely followed by the standard gamble (which is, however, more complex to administer to the lay public). The category method was both less reliable and less valid than either of the former.[9] Again he found a substantial variation, however, in the seriousness with which the various disease states in this

9 Validity (the extent to which the index measures what is purports to measure) was tested by correlating the second two measures with the standard gamble index. Reliability (the extent to which the same subjects assign the same numbers to the same states a second time around) was tested by replicating questions in an ostensibly different form and also by a one-year follow-up test.

TABLE 11

Index scores obtained by time trade-off method (0 = death, 1 = perfect health)

| Judge | Health States | | | | |
	Home Confinement for T.B.	Sanatorium Confinement for T.B.	Kidney Transplant	Home Dialysis	Hospital Dialysis
1	0.61	0.02	0.61	0.55	0.10
2	0.47	0.50	0.94	0.39	0.40
3	0.33	–	0.85	0.61	0.50
4	0.50	0.67	0.96	0.93	0.80
5	0.86	0.75	0.78	0.88	0.80
6	0.50	0.00	0.88	0.05	0.10
7	0.46	0.25	0.91	0.86	0.80
8	0.12	0.11	0.63	0.55	0.38
9	0.81	0.11	1.00	0.97	0.99
10	0.71	0.25	0.84	0.63	0.50
11	0.88	1.00	0.93	0.80	0.92
Mean Score	0.57	0.37	0.85	0.66	0.57

SOURCE: Torrance (1970), Appendix 1, Exhibit 9).

second experiment were regarded by respondents, partly due perhaps to the judges making their own future interpretation of the disabilities of each of the described states of health according to their knowledge but partly due no doubt to their different values.

VALUES, ARBITERS, AND CULTURE

Both with professional and collective decision-making we are confronted not only by the bewildering array of possible approaches discussed above, but also by the necessity of resolving an old problem of political philosophy: whose values shall count? How are conflicts between values to be decided? In medicine, individual patients have, at least in part, surrendered their rights (if they ever had them to surrender!) to different sets of persons and for different reasons. First, they have surrendered the responsibility both for professional judgments and some value judgments to the clinicians. This is the heart of the doctor-patient relationship: a relationship based on trust, especially the trust of the patient that the doctor will interpret his (the patient's) interests as his conscientious agent because the patient is usually ignorant about the natural history of a disease, will have limited vicarious experience of similar cases to his and, *in extremis*, is in no position to make any decisions about anything. As we have seen in earlier chapters, this is the fundamental rock upon which the traditional separation of 'demand' and 'supply' founders. Normatively, we cannot escape the fact that patients are, on the whole, willing to surrender substantial areas of discretion: their values are replaced by the doctors'.

Secondly, because of the complex patterns of the spillovers between sick persons and the rest of society, much of the management of health services and closely related activities lies with non-profit organizations and government. Decisions about which programs are to be funded and which not, about the size of the army of medical manpower, about the distribution of services between regions and households, etc., all these are decisions taken by *agents* of the citizen-voter. Of course, many such decisions are constrained by market-type pressures and some government intentions doubtless get frustrated. Nevertheless, with the removal of the traditional liberal sources of values – consumers in myriad mostly individual-specific decisions – the problem has to be confronted about the best source of values to replace them. Whose values shall count and for what purposes?

The problem is a real one for we know that values vary a good deal among the population. We have already seen from the results of the work of Torrance and Wolfson that different attitudes exist to given conditions, even among relatively homogenous groups, such as doctors. The notion of an 'improvement' in health is thus not a given and constant. As Brook (1973) remarked in a discussion of Chen's (1973) paper: 'Raven did a study on fractured hips and congenital hip problems on Indians. They were treated so they could walk, like a white population. But the Navajo's most important problem is squatting, and by having the hip fixed so he could walk, he couldn't squat. That did a tremendous amount of harm.' The evidence on the submerged part of the 'iceberg' of sickness is eloquent testimony to the fact that many people have serious and treatable illness but 'live' with it, not contacting the medical services. Neither the type of disorder, nor its seriousness by objective medical standards (e.g., prognosis), differentiates effectively between people who 'feel' sick and those who do not (Pearse and Crocker, 1949). In the remainder of this chapter we turn briefly to some of the sociological results that have a bearing on the question of the cultural and social determinants of attitudes to sickness.

Zola's (1966) perceptive discussion noted the inverse correlation between the perceived significance of a disability or symptom and its prevalence and the positive correlation between significant and dominant cultural values:

when the abberation is fairly widespread, this, in itself, might constitute a reason for its not being considered 'symptomatic' or unusual. Among many Mexican-Americans in the Southwestern United States, diarrhea, sweating, and coughing are every-day experiences, while among certain groups of Greeks trachoma is almost universal. Even with our own society, Koos has noted that, although lower back pain is a quite common condition among lower-class women, it is not considered symptomatic of any disease or disorder but part of their expected everyday existence. For the population where the particular condition is ubiquitous, the condition is perceived as the normal state. This does not mean that it is considered 'good' (although instances have been noted where not having the endemic condition was considered abnormal). For example, Ackerknecht (1947) noted that pinto (dichromic spirochetosis), a skin disease, was so common among some South American tribes that the few single men who were not suffering from it were regarded as pathological to the degree of being excluded from marriage. Rather, he says, 'it is natural and inevitable and thus to be ignored as being of no consequence. But the 'symptom' or condition is omnipresent (it always was and always will be) there simply exists for such populations or cultures no frame of reference according to which it could be considered a deviation.' (Zola, 1966, 617-18)

Illustrating the positive correlation, Zola argues that it is the 'fit' of certain signs with a society's major values that account for the attention they receive.

Tiredness, for example, is a physical sign which is not only ubiquitous but a correlate of a vast number of disorders. Yet amongst a group of the author's students who kept a calendar noting all bodily states and conditions, tiredness, though often recorded, was rarely cited as a cause for concern. Attending school and being among peers who stressed the importance of hard work and achievement, almost as an end in itself, tiredness, rather than being an indication of something being wrong was instead positive proof that they were doing right. If they were tired, it must be because they had been working hard. In such a setting tiredness would rarely, in itself, be either a cause for concern, a symptom, or a reason for action or seeking medical aid. On the other hand, where arduous work is not gratifying in and of itself, tiredness would more likely be a matter for concern and perhaps medical attention.

Also illustrative of this process are the divergent perceptions of those bodily complaints often referred to as 'female troubles.' Nausea is a common and treatable concomitant of pregnancy, yet Margaret Meade (1950) records no morning sickness among the Arapesh; her data suggest that this may be related to the almost complete denial that a child exists, until shortly before birth. In a Christian setting, where the existence of life is dated from conception, nausea becomes the external sign, hope and proof that one is pregnant. Thus in the

United States, this symptom is not only quite widespread but is also an expected and almost welcome part of pregnancy. A quite similar phenomenon is the recognition of dysmenorrhea. While Arapesh women reported no pain during menstruation, quite the contrary is reported in the United States. (*ibid.*, 618-19)

Zola found, in a study of Italian and Irish patients, that the same disease produced marked different ethnic perceptions. Different thresholds of pain tolerance, expectation, and acceptance have been widely noted. Zborowski (1952) has noted that pains of childbirth are not accepted in the US and means are used to alleviate it. In Poland it is not only expected but accepted and steps are not taken to relieve it. In fact, it seems that it is the attitude to pain that varies rather than the threshold (Hardy, Wolff, and Goodell 1952). Zborowski found that Jews and Italians were more emotional in their response to pain compared with the relative stoic Irish and 'Old Americans.' Within these broad attitudes, however, Italians are more concerned with the immediacy of the pain sensation (and hence have readier resort to analgesics) than Jews who tend more to emphasize the symptomatic and prognostic meaning of pain and worry about the underlying disease, preferring to suffer (e.g., to avoid possible habit-forming consequences of taking analgesics). The Italian, being more 'present-orientated' has a less sceptical attitude towards his physician's skills than the 'future-orientated' Jews. 'Old Americans' try not to 'make a fuss' about pain, do not like 'being a nuisance to the doctor.' Like the Irish, they need to be specific about the location of pain. Like the Jews, they are 'future-orientated.' These attitudes can, of course, be related to social and economic heritages, cultural influences in childhood upbringing and related social pressures on adult life and, although one should not assume any homogeneity in attitudes within the types reported on, the evidence does indicate that basic values do indeed differ in the population.

It has been noted that concern with health is typically high only when it interferes with daily activity and ability to be independent of others.[10] This supports the basic soundness of the indicators defined in terms of ability to function physically. But it also implies that attitudes to health, and the relative values placed upon different dimensions of handicap, will vary according to individuals' life-styles, jobs, etc. In a real sense, the one-legged professor is less handicapped than the one-legged footballer; the deaf composer more handicapped than the deaf machine-tool operator; the blind painter than the blind musician; the blind painter than the deaf (mindful of Beethoven) musician.

10 Apple (1960) found that whether or not an experience is interpreted by a lay person as a symptom of disease depends on (i) its novelty, and (ii) the extent to which it interferes with ordinary activities. See also Baumann (1961), and Twaddle (1969).

The social, as compared with the biophysical, meaning of illness has been developed principally by Parsons (1951, 1964) and Freidson (1970). Freidson, for example, illustrates an expanded version of Parsons' classification of social attitudes and sick roles as shown in Table 12. These attitudes will, of course, affect the weights placed upon different kinds of disability. We have to ask: are the kinds of weights implied by Table 12 the kind that are really wanted to be reflected in public policy in the health field? In particular, since attaching stigma to some sickness or, indeed, to patients' attitudes to their disability, is not the prerogative of medical people, we have the question of the appropriate role for doctors to play, outside the consulting room, in the setting of values. Koos (1954) found that the lower a person's social class, the less the tendency to consider a given list of symptoms important enough to seek medical attention.

Of particular relevance in the context of the standard gamble approach is the fact that individuals' attitudes to risk vary. While economists have tended to focus on attitudes to risk in the theory of the firm and portfolio investment and, largely because of their concentration on the pure theory, have produced few settled conclusions even regarding how risk-preference or aversion varies with income, it would plainly be an uncomfortable position to hold that all attitudes are the same when both introspection and the casual evidence of our senses denies that this is the case. In health care, religion plainly has a role: at least some who have no faith in an after life exhibit, it has been alleged, a much stronger aversion to the risk of death than is the mode in a basically Christian society. There has, unfortunately, been no study of doctors' attitudes to risk or of the calculations and strategies actually adopted in clinical practice. Indirectly however, we may infer from behaviour that attitudes vary substantially: hospitals vary enormously in the percentage of normal appendixes removed and the size of peptic ulcers operated upon. They also vary greatly according to their rates of prescription of antibacterials in cases of uncomplicated inguinal hernias (where with high standards of hygene and asepsis they are scarcely necessary at all) and – perhaps more disturbingly – they also vary widely in cases of complex herniorrhaphy with its higher risks of infection. Mechanic (1968) argues that the extent to which a doctor is 'conservative' or not in his approach to risks not only depends on his education but a variety of social factors affecting medical practice. It is, therefore, not to be wondered at that different attitudes to risk may help account, even if they will not entirely account, for some of the apparent differences in priority among disease found by, for example, Wolfson and Torrance above.

Several studies (e.g., Friedsam and Martin, 1963; Streib, Suchman, and Phillips, 1958) have shown that doctors' perceptions of ill-health are not in general the same as patients', with the doctors' views based more on 'objective'

TABLE 12

Types of deviance for which the individual is not held responsible, by imputed legitimacy and seriousness (contemporary American middle class societal reaction)

Imputed seriousness	Illegitimate (stigmatized)	Conditionally legitimate	Unconditionally legitimate
Minor deviation	Cell 1 'Stammer' Partial suspension of some ordinary obligations; few or no new privileges; adoption of a few new obligations	Cell 2 'A cold' Temporary suspension of few ordinary obligations; temporary enhancement of ordinary privileges. Obligation to get well	Cell 3 'Pockmarks' No special change in obligations or in privileges
Serious deviation	Cell 4 'Epilepsy' Suspension of some ordinary obligations; adoption of new obligations; few or no new privileges	Cell 5 'Pneumonia' Temporary release from ordinary obligations; addition to ordinary privileges. Obligation to co-operate and seek help in treatment	Cell 6 'Cancer' Permanent suspension of many ordinary obligations; marked addition to privileges

SOURCE: Freidson (1970, 239)

symptoms and prognoses and the patients' tending to correlate with other variables such as psycho-social measures of 'happiness' or anomie. Such differences are, of course, again likely to be reflected in the weights assigned to disability states by different individuals. But it is also clear from the results of economic experiments that there is no homogeneity within groups such as 'physicians' or the 'lay public.'

While it is not our task here to *explain* those value attitudes to health care that vary systematically with observable data (such as ethnicity, social class) clearly they must be taken account of at the very least in the intimacy of the relationship between doctor and patient. And if we are not, on the one hand, to dismiss the idea of constructing health indexes as hopelessly subjective from the beginning or, on the other, to impose an unduly rigid set of values on paternalistic, or whatever, grounds, then some way must be found of building indicators that either avoids arbitrariness by using those values that are commonly shared (if they exist) or is sufficiently sensitive to incorporate important variations.

WHOSE VALUES?

If values are as embodied in health status measurement as we have argued, and inherently so, and if, as appears to be the case, values are not identically shared by individuals in the community, what should be done?

Our analysis suggests two answers. First, the necessity for having to make value judgments should be fairly and squarely faced up to. By systematically exposing the points at which values come in, we hope, in the present chapter, to have simplified this task. Once in the open, value differences, as a reason for reaching different conclusions about priorities, can be identified and argued about.

The second answer relates to those whose values are to count. In Ontario, as in most other developed societies, the responsibility for making value judgments has been delegated to policy-makers. These, at the highest levels, are ministers of the government. At the everyday level, at which policy really gets worked out, they are administrators and professional people in health care agencies of a variety of different kinds. Potentially, we could include the general public or panels of the public as a further source of values (in addition of course to the important role, with which we are not here much concerned, they play as patients when it comes to decisions about the management of specific cases).

The problem is analogous to the constitutional question in political philosophy concerning who should have what rights. There seem to be two broad alternatives. One is that the right árbiters are those who have been placed in the position of arbiter by a legitimate procedure (e.g., by being elected, appointed by those who have been elected, or who are 'trustworthy,' etc.). The other is that the right arbiters are those whose judgments produce what are agreed to be the right results, or the best results under the circumstances when there is agreement not to change the circumstances.

The difficulty with the procedural argument is that we tend to judge the legitimacy of a procedure by the kinds of result it produces. That leaves us essentially with a criterion that judges both the arbiters *and* the procedure by results. If, then, we find ourselves unhappy with, say, the area disposition of health care resources in the province, we may wish to change either the arbiters or the procedure as well. Either task is facilitated by having the elements of decisions clear. Thus, whether we agree that doctors should principally make one set of decisions, or ministry officials another, will depend upon the outcomes of those decisions as judged by those affected by them.

Health policy, like all policy, is messy and tentative, and made under conditions of vast ignorance. The values it embodies are likewise. A rational objective for those wanting a little more efficiency and a little more fairness in the system cannot be to specify in detail who it is that shall decide and what criteria he shall use. Rather, the objective must be to make the general basis for decisions clearer, so that the sources of error may, perhaps, be more clearly seen by all, and to use any of the procedures, pressures and means that are available in society, to bring actual decisions, and the values embodied in them, into line with the desired decisions.

It is for this reason that we cannot specify whose values should be embodied. We must grope and experiment until a reasonable approximation to the desired outcome, whatever it may be, is evolved. One such source of experimental variation is in the values embodied in the output of the health services. The experiment is, of course, everlasting, because the desired results are also changing and evolving.

Since the uses to which health status measures will be put are not thought of as normally containing patient-specific decisions but, rather, concern regional comparisons, or comparisons of treatment outcomes, or comparisons of the outcomes of programs of different sizes, the subtlest and most personal questions of value in health care do not arise. What opinion among index researchers seems to be settling on is the notion of a *representative* weight, typically the average, where the choice of weight is normally distributed about a mean. Both Torrance and Wolfson adopted this approach. Its pragmatic justification is obvious. According to the arguments above, its ethical justificacation will depend upon the acceptability of the consequences of using it.

We should emphasize what has been briefly mentioned in the preceding paragraph: although there is doubtless much to be said for encouraging physicians to think quite specifically about patient outcomes, and although (as we shall see later) there are applications of health status measurement in monitoring quality of care, the principal context in which the measure would be used would *not* include a kind of 'big brother' controlling of individual members of the medical profession as they apply their knowledge and experience to individual patients. The object is *not* to specify in detail what physicians in their daily practice should be doing. Rather, it is to help in deciding broader allocation questions relating to the resources that are going to be made available – including the number and/or location of physicians, the amount of support facilities, etc. These do, of course, constrain the individual physician but the general objective is so to organize the resource constraints that they appropriately reflect local needs and medical technology. Within these constraints, the professional has, as now, to exercise his or her professional judgment about how best to allocate the resources at his or her disposal.

It should also be emphasized that the values embodied in a macro index of community health status, or in more micro measures designed for specific purposes, need neither be the same nor, in particular, are they to be regarded as fixed and immutable for all time. As the problems change, as perceptions of problems change, as technology changes, and as the degree of success in combatting ill-health among sub-classifications of the community progresses, so will the relative importance attached to particular kinds of disability, particular causes of impairment of function, and particular client groups.

It is precisely to aid the, ultimately political, choice of priorities that the information about ability to function is designed. And while there are undoubtedly value judgments of our first type (on p. 58) involved in the selection of dimensions such as those in the activities of daily living schedule used by Katz (see above, p. 55) the controversy is likely to be less strong about these than about the relative importance to be attached to one dimension rather than another. Indeed, it is highly likely that very speedy agreement will be reached that these dimensions are, indeed, generally relevant, that they should be supplemented by dimensions of pain and anxiety and that they should also be given a duration in time. *How* these dimensions are best measured is largely, if not as we have seen entirely, a question for 'experts.' *And this is all that need be decided* prior to designing and conducting a community survey. The other values, and how they ought to change as circumstances change, are essentially matters concerning the *interpretation* of the results. As we have said above, the validity of this interpretation must ultimately be tested by the general acceptability of its consequences in terms of decisions taken (or not taken!). As we hope to show in the final chapter, however, there is some guidance which can be given and which makes the agnosticism that seems inherent in this approach more apparent than real.

6
Uses and users of health measures

Although the preceding chapter has drawn on a variety of different studies from different countries and designed for different purposes, our emphasis there was on the *construction* of the measures. In this chapter, we turn the emphasis around and, without inquiring too deeply into methods of construction, look more closely at how the measures that may be derived can be used and for whom they may be useful. It will doubtless have become clear by now that the 'output' or 'outcome' orientation of health measurement is so fundamental a perspective that it is, in truth, all-pervading in any health service and ought to be the centre of focus for any who make decisions which may ultimately affect the health of individuals, from the minister of health at one extreme to the most junior qualified nurse at the other.

We shall, perforce, have to resort to illustrations. But to give them some institutional reality and to locate them in time and space, we shall draw them from the province of Ontario. For some purposes, of course, such as those related to inter-provincial comparisons or where national programs or data collection potentially have important provincial implications (as has, for example, the Canada Health Survey) we shall have to look at the wider Canadian community.

The principal user of health measures we shall term, in a general way, the 'health care administrator' in Donabedian's sense (Donabedian, 1973) of a hypothetical figure: an amalgam of all persons in the medical care system who are called upon to make decisions and to monitor processes in the organization and delivery of medical care. Our approach is similar to that of the Ontario Council of Health (1975): 'the first requirement of the health statistics system is to provide data for use in the planning, operation, and evaluation of health services and programs in Ontario' (21). This chapter is not, then, a manual for specific kinds of practitioner or administrator. But it is intended to focus a general way of thinking on selected examples so that the imaginative and intelligent 'administrator,' whatever his seniority and whatever the range of his responsibilities, can see how a clear perception of ends and means is not mere pie-in-the-sky armchair taxonomizing but actually helpful in concrete problem-solving.

In this chapter we shall look at five examples of the way in which health measurement has been or could be used in Ontario: (*a*) Interregional comparisons (international, interprovincial, and intraprovincial); (*b*) research priorities; (*c*) monitoring performance and quality of care; (*d*) utilization and distributional effects; (*e*) cost-effectiveness.

INTERREGIONAL COMPARISONS

There is an overwhelming case, when making *international* comparisons, for minimizing the intrusion of value questions of the sort discussed at length in chapter five, for the variance in the significance of ill health, and of its dimensions, is normally to be expected to be a good deal larger between countries than within a country and, typically, there would be less consensus about relative priorities at the margin among countries of varying degrees of development. In any case, at this level, the rudimentary comparison of mortality rates (including causes of death) and longevity is the most that can realistically be hoped for, particularly since for many poor countries, the effort required even to collect statistics of the most primitive variables is enormous and the data thus procured are not always of the highest degree of reliability.

More detail and sophistication are possible, however, in comparisons of countries at similar stages of development and sharing similar cultural values. One recent example of an *ad hoc* comparison between similar countries is Cochrane's comparison of the ostensible effectiveness of the health services in five European countries, the USA, and Canada (Cochrane, 1975).

Some of Cochrane's data are shown in Table 13. The value of indexes of this kind, provided that the comparisons are between broadly similar countries in terms of their values, wealth, and available technology, is basically two-fold. First, a broad picture is obtained of the relative standing of one's own country *vis-a-vis* others in terms of some indicators judged to be important. Second a picture, again broad, is given as to how these 'results' are associated with different degrees of resource availability. Of course the picture is a partial one. The mortality data are highly imperfect measures of health status (though death is undoubtedly a limitation of function). The column averaging the rank orders

TABLE 13

Ranking of seven countries by selected indicators (1971)

Country	Mortality rank order							
	Peri-natal	Infant	Ma-ternal	Males 34-44	Males 45-54	Females 35-44	Females 45-54	Average
Sweden	1	1	1	2	1	2	1	1.3
Netherlands	2	2	2	1	2	1	2	1.7
England and Wales	4	3	2	3	4	5	6	3.9
Canada	3	4	4	5	5	4	4	4.1
Italy	7	7	7	4	3	3	3	4.9
France	5	5	6	6	6	6	5	5.6
USA	6	6	5	7	7	7	7	6.4

SOURCE: Derived from Tables II, III, and V in Cochrane (1975).

of mortality rates is a crude (quick and dirty) method of combining the mortality data. The causal relationships between mortality and the provision rankings in the five columns on the right hand side of the tables are not known. Nevertheless, despite these manifest shortcomings, such comparisons have the great merit of pointing, sometimes dramatically, to important questions – questions whose answers, of course, depend upon much more detailed investigations. The questions are prompted by the similarities and differences observed.

Some of the more obvious questions raised by Table 13 are: (a) Why does the USA, which ranks high in terms of its spending, its physician/population ratio, and its hospitalization rate, rank so low in the mortality rate league? (b) What accounts, in particular, for the enormous difference in mortality between Sweden and the USA, which have an almost identical rate of hospital admission? (c) Why is it that Canada and Britain, with nearly identical experience of mortality, differ so markedly in the resources expended on health services? (d) Why are Italy's adult mortality rates so out of line with those associated with childbirth? (e) What accounts for the consistently good performance of Sweden and the Netherlands? (f) How come that Britain, after nearly thirty years of 'free' health care, not only spends less than anyone else but come into the top three as far as 'results' are concerned, contrary to all the predictions of the deprecators of 'socialized' medicine? (g) Is Canada getting value for her high level of spending and, in particular, her high rate of hospital admission?

TABLE 13, *continued*

Other rankings				
Health Expenditure as % GNP	Physicians per 10,000 pop.	Nurses per 10,000 pop.	General hospital rates per 10,000 pop.	Hospital admissions per 10,000 pop.
3	4	3	1	3
4	6	2	3	6
7	7	5	7	4
2	3	1	2	1
6	5	6	6	7
5	1	7	4	5
1	2	4	5	2

Posing such questions leads, of course, to this more precise formulation and research into the answers. One particular kind of research prompted by considerations such as these involves an examination of the way other countries have tackled problems. Given the substantial differences in different countries' experiences, history, modes of organizing and delivering health services, conventions of clinical practice, environment, and so on, the rich possibilities inherent in such studies are probably not exploited as fully as they should be. Even skilled veterans at this international game, such as Odin Anderson, tend to come to conclusions that are, for all their plausibility, still disturbingly general: 'the dominant reason why the Swedish mortality rates are lower than in any state in the United States is a high minimum standard of living for everyone and a cultural homogeneity of life styles of sanitation and cleanliness ... the elimination of poverty in the United States in the sense true for Sweden would be more likely to bring mortality rates closer to Sweden than a policy limited to health services only' (Anderson, 1972, 158). Such a conclusion can be inferred by investigating cause and age of death and associating death at certain ages and from certain causes with, say, 'poverty.' It yet remains, however, for someone to investigate in detail the precise empirical relationships between poverty, life style, etc. and mortality in international studies. Yet the data, or reasonable proxies for the correctly specified variables, commonly exist in most developed countries in basically comparable form, even if there currently exists no ready way of exploring these factors in their relationship with a true measure of ill health.

Interesting and important though the questions prompted by such comparisons are (especially when they seek to *explain* the differences observed) they are not, of course, directly relevant in the planning processes of any single country though they may point the directions in which policy might be directed. But as soon as we pass from the international to the intranational level, the indicators take on a whole new significance at either a federal or a provincial level. Since society has objectives for its health services that are couched in terms of their geographic provision, area information on health status takes on the status of a policy variable and resource provision becomes an instrument of policy.

It has become conventional to distinguish two basic criteria for area allocations of health care resources: demand and need. In delivery systems where utilization is largely divorced from payment by patients, as in Ontario, the procedure cannot rely upon area expenditures as indicators of relative demands. Instead, focus tends to be upon utilization itself. Unfortunately, as we have seen above, demand as utilization is not independent of supply: for example, areas of equal utilization may have differing underlying morbidity patterns — which may not even become reflected in queues, if queues develop. This interdependence, sometimes referred to in connection with hospitals as Roemer's law (Roemer, 1961)[1] really destroys the usefulness of demand (or excess demand) as a behavioural indicator of resource allocation, since in health care demand is revealed, via the doctor-patient relationship, only in relative terms, that is, relative to supply, and increasing supply instead of reducing excess demand, may *increase* demand with excess demand either rising or falling. It should be added that demand studies are not without importance in *behavioural analysis*: viz, *explaining* differences in utilization rates or *predicting* future utilization rates. As a basis for a normative criterion for area allocation they are, however, not merely inadequate alone but can be quite misleading.

In addition to the all-pervading influence of existing supply on utilization rates, we have argued above that the spillover effects of good and ill health make demand less relevant, even were Roemer's law not to operate and even were it to be the case that physicians as agents of their patients *perfectly* represented their interests. Although conceptually the implications of the spillover effects (especially the humanitarian spillovers) derive from the same 'neo-classical' set of ideas that provided rigorous justifications for 'laissez-faire,' in practice they imply the necessity of collective action based on an interpretation not only of patients' demands but the *community's* demand or, as it is more conventionally termed, need.

1 As we have seen earlier, Evans (1974) has found interdependence to be inherent in fee-per-service systems. But the effect has been noted also under salaried and capitation systems (e.g., Airth and Newell, 1962; Culyer and Cullis, 1976).

At the crudest level, criteria based upon need are indistinguishable from similarly crude criteria based upon demand. Thus the initial formula for allocating funds to regions in England and Wales was based upon regional population and could equally be interpreted as a crude demand or crude need indicator. In any event (i.e., whichever interpretation one accepts) its introduction in the early 1970s marked a substantial improvement on the previous convention which amounted essentially to the preceding year's budget plus some small negotiable increase: a procedure which had done very little to alter the distribution of resource inherited from pre-NHS days (Cooper and Culyer, 1972).

Studies which attempt to measure need in more sophisticated ways than head-counting are, however, exceedingly scarce. The nearest thing to such a measure for Ontario is in Wolfson's 1974 study whose methodology was described in outline in chapter five above. Aside from this, the only routinely published statistics relating to need for areas within the province are crude death rates, perinatal mortality and deaths by cause and sex (others, such as life expectancy at selected ages, could be obtained from census data, but are not routinely produced). This situation will have to be improved with the growth of district health councils if they are to discharge properly the duties placed upon them by the provincial minister of health.

Wolfson, it will be recalled, used the 'standard gamble' method to calculate weights of severity to be attached to 59 diseases and subsequently extrapolated them to over 223 diseases. By applying these weights to OHIP claims data and hospital separation data and dividing by the population at risk, two updated indexes were computed. The results, by county, for October 1972 are shown in Table 14, together with crude death rates and perinatal death rates for 1973 (from Figure 7). Table 15 shows the proportional deviation of each of these four indicators from the provincial average.

Interpreting the indexes as descriptive measures, possibly indicating priority areas warranting more detailed investigation, several questions are raised. One is not immediately apparent from the tables and derives from the small number of deaths occurring in some areas. This is particularly applicable to perinatal mortality and, for this reason, the average of two years was taken.

Another problem arises from the way the health indexes were constructed. In Table 15, the low value of the hospital health index for Glengarry is remarkable in itself, and even more remarkable in the light of the extremely high mortality rates there. It is probably explained by the fact that the index is derived from hospital separations data and most of those from Glengarry who are hospitalized outside the county. As we shall see in the next chapter, interpreting these health measures, in the context of the effects that resource provision may have, is not a straightforward matter.

TABLE 14

Health status measures for Ontario 1972-3, by county

County	Wolfson's hospital health index	Wolfson's claims health index	Crude mortality rate per 1000	Perinatal mortality rate per 1000 births (inc. stillbirths) average of 1972-3
Algoma	3.96	53	6.42	18.3
Brant	5.83	84	8.77	20.6
Bruce	3.40	66	10.21	14.7
Cochrane	3.66	55	7.57	24.7
Dufferin	5.01	38	9.01	31.8
Dundas	4.32	87	10.96	24.0
Durham	3.38	48	7.96	17.4
Elgin	4.48	69	9.52	19.4
Essex	3.57	75	8.13	22.1
Frontenac	6.79	89	7.30	18.4
Glengarry	0.95	55	12.32	32.0
Grenville	1.71	60	9.10	24.0
Grey	5.52	82	10.46	21.7
Haldimand	3.29	80	8.77	25.1
Haliburton	3.98	47	11.17	29.9
Halton	3.78	48	4.92	16.8
Hastings	5.15	83	9.03	17.8
Huron	5.07	76	10.85	16.8
Kenora	2.84	44	8.44	21.0
Kent	4.65	70	8.91	22.0
Lambton	3.93	68	8.04	22.9
Lanark	5.71	88	11.45	26.1
Leeds	4.29	65	10.12	22.8
Lennox and Addington	2.12	45	7.88	21.4
Manitoulin	2.04	54	11.80	17.9
Middlesex	7.10	79	7.33	16.7
Muskoka	3.23	52	10.57	24.0
Niagara	4.89	72	7.99	21.2
Nipissing	3.86	57	7.68	23.1
Norfolk	3.72	67	10.30	23.5
Northumberland	1.60	60	9.45	22.0
Ontario	3.18	43	6.74	19.8
Ottawa	2.76	61	6.85	19.6
Oxford	5.77	76	9.03	19.2
Parry Sound	4.50	81	10.23	20.6
Peel	2.26	28	3.94	15.7
Perth	4.34	59	9.51	23.7
Peterborough	6.19	76	8.94	24.6

TABLE 14, *continued*

Health status measures for Ontario 1972-3, by county

County	Wolfson's hospital health index	Wolfson's claims health index	Crude mortality rate per 1000	Perinatal mortality rate per 1000 births (inc. stillbirths) average of 1972-3
Prescott	2.55	54	7.78	29.7
Prince Edward	1.42	77	11.84	25.3
Rainy River	5.38	62	9.22	30.0
Renfrew	3.86	55	7.92	21.9
Russell	N.A.	84	9.48	25.3
Simcoe	4.34	40	8.92	18.6
Stormont	7.13	68	8.71	23.5
Sudbury	2.47	48	5.47	21.6
Thunder Bay	4.79	56	9.05	16.2
Timiskaming	3.88	57	9.82	26.1
Toronto	5.22	40	7.08	18.3
Victoria	6.59	77	11.39	16.3
Waterloo	2.79	59	6.29	19.3
Wellington	4.24	61	7.61	19.7
Wentworth	6.17	78	7.75	17.8
York	5.03	40	7.59	18.7
PROVINCE	4.46	56	7.54	19.5

TABLE 15

Health status measures for Ontario 1972-3, by county, as proportionate deviation from provincial average

County	Wolfson's hospital health index	Wolfson's claims health index	Crude mortality rate per 1000	Perinatal mortality rate per 1000 births (inc. stillbirths average of 1972-3
Algoma	−0.11	−0.05	−0.15	−0.16
Brant	0.31	0.50	0.16	0.06
Bruce	−0.24	0.18	0.35	−0.25
Cochrane	−0.18	−0.02	0.0	0.27
Dufferin	0.12	−0.32	0.19	0.63
Dundas	−0.03	0.55	0.45	0.23
Durham	−0.24	−0.14	0.06	−0.11
Elgin	0.0	0.23	0.26	−0.01
Essex	−0.20	0.34	0.08	0.13

TABLE 15, *continued*

Health status measures in Ontario 1972-3, by county, as proportionate deviation from provincial average

County	Wolfson's hospital health index	Wolfson's claims health index	Crude mortality rate per 1000	Perinatal mortality rate per 1000 births (inc. stillbirths) average of 1972-3
Frontenac	0.52	0.59	−0.03	−0.06
Glengarry	−0.79	−0.02	0.63	0.64
Grenville	−0.52	0.07	0.21	0.23
Grey	0.24	0.46	0.39	0.11
Haldimand	−0.26	0.43	0.16	0.29
Haliburton	−0.11	−0.16	0.48	0.53
Halton	−0.15	−0.14	−0.35	−0.14
Hastings	0.15	0.48	0.20	−0.09
Huron	0.14	0.36	0.44	−0.14
Kenora	−0.36	−0.21	0.12	0.08
Kent	0.04	0.25	0.18	0.13
Lambton	−0.12	0.21	0.07	0.17
Lanark	0.28	0.57	0.52	0.34
Leeds	−0.04	0.16	0.34	0.20
Lennox and Addington	−0.52	−0.20	0.05	0.10
Manitoulin	−0.54	−0.04	0.56	−0.08
Middlesex	0.59	0.41	−0.03	−0.14
Muskoka	−0.28	−0.07	0.40	0.23
Niagara	0.10	0.29	0.06	0.09
Nipissing	−0.13	0.02	0.02	0.18
Norfolk	−0.17	0.20	0.37	0.21
Northumberland	−0.64	0.07	0.25	0.13
Ontario	−0.29	−0.23	−0.11	−0.02
Ottawa	−0.38	0.09	−0.09	0.01
Oxford	0.29	0.36	0.20	−0.02
Parry Sound	0.01	0.45	0.37	0.06
Peel	−0.49	−0.50	−0.48	−0.19
Perth	−0.03	0.05	0.26	0.22
Peterborough	0.39	0.36	0.19	0.26
Prescott	−0.43	−0.04	0.03	0.52
Prince Edward	−0.68	0.38	0.57	0.30
Rainy River	0.21	0.11	0.22	0.54
Renfrew	−0.13	−0.02	0.05	0.12
Russell	N.A.	0.50	0.26	0.30
Simcoe	−0.03	−0.29	0.18	−0.05
Stormont	0.60	0.21	0.16	0.21

TABLE 15, *continued*

Health status measures in Ontario 1972-3, by county, as proportionate deviation from provincial average

County	Wolfson's hospital health index	Wolfson's claims health index	Crude mortality rate per 1000	Perinatal mortality rate per 1000 births (inc. stillbirths) average of 1972-3
Sudbury	−0.45	−0.14	−0.27	0.11
Thunder Bay	0.07	0.0	0.20	−0.17
Timiskaming	−0.13	0.01	0.30	0.34
Toronto	0.17	−0.29	−0.06	−0.06
Victoria	0.48	0.38	0.51	−0.14
Waterloo	−0.37	0.05	−0.17	−0.01
Wellington	−0.05	0.09	0.01	0.01
Wentworth	0.38	0.39	0.03	−0.09
York	0.13	−0.29	0.01	−0.04

The use of crude death rates is not a reliable indicator of the relative life chances of an average person in different counties, since it fails to account, in particular, for the age and sex characteristics of county populations. As a rough indication of the severity of health problems, on the assumption that death is equally undesirable for an old as for a young person, male or female, it is less objectionable. The causes of death, like the disease composition of the Wolfson indexes, are of course important further descriptions to which we shall turn briefly later.

Finally, we should recall from chapter five that the 'degree of measurability' in the health indexes is not the same as that in the mortality indexes. Thus, while it is perfectly correct to say that the death rate in Timiskaming is twice that in Halton, it is not correct to say that Essex is twice as healthy as Stormont.[2] The reason for this is that the standard gamble method of weighting sickness incidents produces an interval scale, not a ratio scale. Thus, we can compare the ratios only of the *differences* between scores or, as in Table 15, the differences expressed as a proportion of the average. Reverting to the illustrative comparison of Essex and Stormont, while the statement that Essex is twice as healthy as Stormont strictly has no meaning at all, the statement that Essex is

2 Wolfson's otherwise excellent discussion of his results slips into this fallacy at times (e.g., Wolfson, 1974, 19). Note that the problem would not arise if the only source of variation were in the number of persons of a given case-severity (this number is measured on a ratio scale) rather than in the number of persons and in case-severity.

twenty per cent better than average and Stormont 60 per cent worse provides a precise statement of the information given us by the Wolfson hospital health index about the relative healthiness of the two counties.

Although not required by the method of constructing the measures, we have for convenience also presented the mortality data in Table 15 as proportionate deviations from the average.

It is perhaps not necessary at this stage to emphasize that the interpretation of the information in Tables 14 and 15 hinges crucially upon the acceptability of the value judgments (weights) used in its construction. Although we have emphasized before that the medical profession is not the only set of persons having claim to competence and legitimacy in assigning weights, one interesting implication of the Wolfson measures is that to the extent that the weights are representative of medical opinion, the consequential implied priorities should correspond to the profession's view. This may also, of course, turn out to lead to satisfactory results as judged by the public.

Again, it should be emphasized that the Wolfson measures are not directly based upon individuals' *ability to function*, though doubtless notions of associated functional ability informed the judgments of his physicians when they assigned the weights to each disease category. The procedure, beginning as it did with disease definitions, effectively precluded, of course, anyone other than a physician from making these judgments.

Most of these inherent limitations again apply if the Wolfson indexes are used to estimate priorities in terms of the definitions of diseases. He found that, for both indexes, the rankings produced by those diseases contributing most to the measure of ill-health were not the same as those having the highest incidence. Rankings based upon the 1972 data in Wolfson's study are shown in Table 16. Although it is not done here, it would be a relatively simple matter to compute the contribution to the total local index score made by specific diseases in each locality: an exercise which would, of course, give a much more informative picture concerning the nature of the problem confronted (or, more precisely, given the process base for the data, *actually being met*) in each locality. Once again, however, distortions in the hospital index due to the existence of concentrations of some specialties in relatively few 'centres of excellence,' would have to be borne in mind when interpreting the results. It would be a relatively simple further extension to compute a 'Q' index (see chapter five) of a rather sophisticated variety using these data, by which deviations from the provincial norm could be calculated.

A principal difficulty noted by Wolfson and frequently encountered by those seeking to use OHIP records as a basis for deriving criteria for evaluating the province's health programs, lies in the inadequacy of the diagnostic information

TABLE 16

Rank order of diseases by incidence and contribution to health measures in Ontario, 1972

	Rank order of diseases			
	Claims health index		Hospital health index	
OHIP code No. of disease	Contribution to index	Incidence	Contribution to index	Incidence
100	1	2	3	4
97	2	1	9	7
21–55	3	6	1	1
99	4	5	2	2
103	5	10	4	6
59	6	3	7	5
189	7	7	11	8
64	8	4	13	12
104	9	9	12	11
145	10	11	5	9
119	11	8	8	3
44	12	13	6	10
80	13	12	10	13

SOURCE: Tables Va and Vb in Wolfson (1974)
NOTES: The diseases represented by OHIP categories are: 21-55 cancers other than leukaemia; 44 leukaemia; 59 diabetes mellitus; 64 other metabolic diseases; e.g., amyloid degeneration of bone, electrolyte imbalance, general metastatic calcification, gout, metabolic disease, necrosis, non-vascular collagen disease, obesity; 80 multiple sclerosis; 97 hypertensive disease; 99 other ischaemic heart disease, e.g., angina, cardiac ischemia, cardiovascular disease, coronary arteriosclerosis, coronary artery narrowing, coronary disease, coronary insufficiency, myocardial ischemia, senile coronary disease; 100 other heart disease, e.g., auricular fibrillation, bradycardia, bundle branch block, cardiac arrest, cardiac asthenia, cardiac asthma, cardiac atrophy, cardiac dyspnea, cardiac oedema, cardiac exhaustion, cardiac insufficiency, cardiovascular oedema, carditis, congestive heart disease, congestive heart failure, endocarditis, heart enlargment, extra systoles, fibroid heart disease, flutter, heart action disorder, heart ascites, heart block, heart irregularity, mitral stenosis, myocardial block, myocarditis, murmur, organic and pulmonary heart disease, paroxysmal tachycardia, pericarditis, Stroke-Adams disease; 103 other cerebro-vascular disease, e.g., aneurysm of meninges, apoplexy, arteriosclerotic encephalopathy, cerebral haemorrhage, cerebral arteriosclerosis, cerebral effusion, cerebral ischemia, cerebral vascular accident, haemiplegia, stroke; 104 arteriosclerosis; 119 asthma; 145 cirrhosis of the liver; 189 rheumatoid arthritis and allied conditions.

written on OHIP claims cards by practitioners (e.g., 40 per cent in the categories 780 and 799: senility and ill-defined symptoms). Since the OHIP claims system is such a potentially rich source of planning information it is of the highest degree of desirability that the information on the cards be both as accurate and as specific as possible. Properly administered, and notwithstanding the limitations we have noted, this information base could, at almost no additional expense, prove to be the envy of almost all other countries – and certainly provide more systematic routine information on patients than is available even in countries such as Britain with a longer tradition of providing comprehensive medical care at public expense.

A further important limitation of data that are based upon process (*viz*; patients treated by 'institutions' such as hospitals or general practices) is that they do not necessarily reflect the underlying need of the relevant community, whether defined geographically or in terms of client groups of other kinds. This arises for two principal reasons. First, persons who are not treated by the 'system' are not recorded in the data. Only if untreated and treated cases bear a constant ratio to one another can the latter be considered a useful indicator either of the former or of the total. Second, which is particularly important in geographical measures, is the difficulty that persons are located according to place of treatment rather than place of residence. While hospital data do include patients' addresses (though these were not used in the Wolfson indexes) the OHIP data do not currently identify patient addresses. This second difficulty could, of course, be resolved by recording them; the first limitation of process-based data is, however, inherent in using such data and can ultimately be overcome only by properly conducted community surveys.

Returning to the interpretation of the indexes in Tables 14 and 15, however, it is not difficult to see that inherent difficulties strongly argue for going a good deal further than relying on existing (institutional) data sources. Some of these difficulties are perfectly general and arise whenever one has more than one index purporting to measure basically the same thing. Others are more fundamental.

Although the *a priori* interpretation of these measures is apparently clear – in Table 14 high values of each measure indicate a worse community health status while in Table 15, negative and positive values indicate respectively better or worse states relative to the average – it is clear that the indicators do not move together precisely. The Spearman correlation coefficient between the proportionate deviations in the hospital index and the claims index in Table 15 is + 0.49, and is statistically highly significant. However, the hospital index is not correlated at all with the crude mortality rate (a county with high general mortality is neither more nor less likely to have a high index of hospital sickness than a county with low crude mortality), while there is even a small negative correlation of – 0.18 between hospital sickness and perinatal mortality (which is statistically significant at the 90 per cent level).

The claims index is positively correlated (0.36) with crude mortality and is statistically highly significant but is not at all correlated with perinatal mortality;

while crude mortality, as is to be expected, is significantly correlated with perinatal mortality (0.37).

This exercise is sufficient to indicate the current difficulty of measuring health status in a region. It focuses attention on the dangers inherent in reliance solely on mortality measures. The results also indicate that the four measures, to the extent that each is considered itself to be an interesting indicator of some dimension(s) of community health, are not measures of the same thing.

In the next chapter we explore in greater detail the association between these health measures, the resources available by county and other socio-economic characteristics of the populations. It is again a point worth repeating that the two Wolfson indexes are each dependent on patients being processed by the health care system; they do not pick up untreated illness or illness where no consultation takes place with a physician. Thus, to the extent that increases in the numbers of physicians and hospital beds per county do not lead to a proportionate reduction in workloads, such increases are to be expected to *increase* the county indexes — just as reductions are expected to reduce them: increased provision of services may lead to an apparent increase in ill-health. Such are the inescapable and paradoxical consequences of indexes that are dependent upon health care *process*. Whether the gain in detail and precision from using process records compensates for the failure of such measures to measure underlying morbidity, which can be measured only by direct sampling and social surveys, is a matter for judgment. Our own view is that though the Wolfson indexes are better than anything else around, their usefulness is much reduced by their dependence upon process and the focus on diagnosis. Such is inevitable with reliance upon existing data sources, which were not designed with health measurement in mind. In the Wolfson indexes, the significance of the personal and social consequences of disease only gets in 'through the back door," so to speak, in the weights, which are simultaneously an amalgam of judgments about the probable consequences of disease, the weights placed on these consequences, the duration of the consequences, and the individual judges' attitudes to the probabilities themselves. It was, of course, to avoid this simultaneous assessment of many diverse factors that the various steps of chapter four and five were spelled out. It is an inherent limitation of using the diagnostic categories of OHIP and hospital separation data, that these distinctions become impossible to consider individually.

It is in this context that the Canada Health Survey scheduled to be undertaken by Statistics Canada beginning in 1978 is to be seen as offering exciting new possibilities, deriving directly from the 'regulatory strategy' of *A New Perspective on the Health of Canadians* (Lalonde 1974). The basic questions to be asked in the survey are 29 in number, each broken down into more specific questions. They follow the broad groupings of human biology, environment, lifestyle, and health care organization, which were identified in *A New Perspective* while some, with which we are particularly concerned here, relate directly to health status.[3]

The principal pieces of information to be sought are: (*a*) functional ability; (*b*) perceived symptoms and disease; (*c*) various bio-physical measurements; (*d*) personal dimensions of mental health; (*e*) social dimensions of mental health.

Of these, some (*a*, some of *b*, *d*, and *e*) are measures of functioning ability or personal comfort, while others are indicative of underlying causes of disability and discomfort or are a basis for prognostication about the likelihood of future disability and discomfort (some of *b*, *c*). It is to be noted that symptoms are an ambiguous category: some may not interfere at all with good health, others may interfere but whether they do so depends upon the individual's lifestyle, some describe clinical characteristics of a disease (which may or may not affect functioning), and have small prognostic value while others may act as warning signals of trouble to come. The specific measures proposed are as follows:

(*a*) *Functional ability*
This, like the British general household survey and the annual health interview survey in the United States, has two principal elements: short-term disability, relating to restrictions of activity, work or school absence and bed confinement within the previous two weeks, and long-standing restrictions, relating to ability to perform daily living activities and restrictions on mobility over the previous twelve months.

The uses which these measures are seen as serving include the fundamental one of providing 'baseline' data on health status where currently none exists, and to monitor it over time; to assess the need for domiciliary and institutional maintenance, and other services and preventive measures; to plan for the employment of the disabled.

(*b*) *Perceived symptoms and diseases*
Again split into short-term and longstanding categories, questions will be asked relating to conditions, accidents and injuries occuring in the previous two weeks and chronic conditions, handicaps and impairments over the previous year, including defects in hearing, vision, dental status, learning difficulties, and mental retardation.

These questions essentially complement those under (*a*) giving some idea of the causes or clinical nature of restrictions of activity. This will enable a

3 The account here is based on Stephens (1976).

comparison to be made between the handicapping conditions of a random sample of the population with those utilizing health service facilities, and will shed light on specific questions relating to, for example, the distribution of dentists or the effectiveness of fluoridation programs.

(c) Bio-physical measures

These measures, in contrast to the self-reported characteristics in (a) and (b) will be based upon measurement by instruments. Measurements to be included are: (i) Canadian home fitness test (pulse rates during and after sub-maximal exercise) for a sub-sample of respondents aged 15 and over; (ii) blood pressure for a sub-sample of respondents aged 5 and over; (iii) per cent body fat (standing height, weight, wrist breadth, upper arm circumference, triceps skinfold, shoulder-elbow length) for a sub-sample aged 5 and over; (iv) height and weight for a sub-sample of respondents of between 1 year and 5 years of age; (v) Haemoglobin and haemocrit to indicate anaemia for a sub-sample aged 15 and over; (vi) creatinine determinations to indicate kidney function for a sub-sample aged 15 and over; (vii) enzyme determinations to indicate liver function. These measures are significant in being a much more ambitious undertaking than any used in the British general household survey, and go beyond the proposals of the OECD health indicators team. Again these measures would complement the functional measures in (a), would provide information on 'positive' health (physical fitness), would provide further indicants of future potential disabling conditions, giving trends over time, and provide follow-up to specific community programs such as the Nutrition Canada survey of anaemia.[4]

(d) Personal dimensions of mental health

Using scales developed elsewhere, the three dimensions here proposed include anxiety and depression, hostility, and personality disorders.

Again the uses of the information include the provision of 'baseline' data where none currently exist, to relate the answers to (a) of underlying causes, and to assess the distribution of needs in relation to the distribution of resources.

(e) Social dimensions of mental health

The dimensions that are currently proposed for measurement include family

---

4 In one study of Lennox and Addington county, rural Frontenac, and Kingston (Law *et al.*, 1973) a clinical examination was included as part of a health status and health service utilization study and it was concluded that 'it contributed little additional information' to self-reported status (p. 23). Unfortunately, details of the 'clinical investigation' were not given in this paper.

functioning, job satisfaction, family-work conflict and alcohol-related problems that are unrelated to physical health.

The uses are seen as essentially the same as those for (*d*), while it is also hoped that some light may be shed on industrial labour relations, sickness absence from work and developments in the nuclear family.

In addition to these questions relating directly to health status, an extensive set of questions relating to the 'health fields' of *A New Perspective* will also be asked. Thus, these will relate to lifestyle (including use of alcohol and tobacco), bio-medical information relating, for example, to immunization status; environmental measures (including, for example, trace elements detected in the blood samples, job stresses); utilization of health services; accessibility of health services (including cost and distance); and basic demographic, socio-economic, and household information. It has yet to be decided whether linkages will be established between the survey and the patients' records via use of insurance numbers. Clearly, for checking the validity of some responses, obtaining better diagnostic information and supplementing utilization data, such a step would be highly desirable. This additional step would also provide direct information about the 'submerged iceberg' of sickness, and provide on a national and provincial scale a continuous monitoring procedure that has hitherto been undertaken in this depth only for shorter periods of time in restricted areas (e.g., the Peckham experiment, see Pearse and Crocker, 1949) apart from the health interview survey of the US National Center for Health Statistics.

Although there exists no general statement describing the underlying philosophy of the Canada Health Survey analogous to the very full OECD discussion, the most significant difference between the two conceptions lies in the fact that the OECD program is hoped to take a *predictive* nature, describing the future expectations of healthfulness of existing populations whereas the Canada Health Survey is more static in design, with its predictive elements only implicitly contained within it in the form of the bio-physical measures. Now, although these latter require a macro-epidemiological model in order for one to make predictions about future health status, future needs, future utilization, etc., it seems preferable to face up squarely to this issue and, in time, to use the data generated by the survey for testing such models. The alternative which seems to be that intended by OECD, is to make predictions about future levels of functioning by extrapolating from disabilities experienced by current age cohorts and adjusting for expected survival rates. The validity and hence the usefulness of this procedure clearly depends upon an unchanging underlying incidence of causative factors relating to lifestyle and exposure to disease-inducing agents. But since there are exogenous changes occurring in these over time, as well as endogenous ones deriving from policy, the Canada Health Survey approach lends itself more effectively to a sophisticated treatment, using epidemiological knowledge already in existence and, in time, adding to that knowledge as relationships emerge from the data themselves.

The breadth of the questions currently proposed in the Survey, however, means that there will be less detailed information on physical ability to function than would be desirable from the point of view of constructing indexes having some sensitivity in measuring degrees of functional ability, and hence its value as a planning aid, or in developing social-epidemiological models, will be restricted as compared with its use in painting a broad picture of trends in health status. This, as well as the fact that it is currently planned only to survey 40,000 individuals in the whole country, with provincial quotas determined by the square root of each province's population, severely limits its usefulness at the provincial level in Ontario and, in particular, its use at the district health council level.

Its broadness is a natural consequence of its close relationship with *A New Perspective* and its design fitting into the 'health field' concepts developed in that document which are intended to show, at a rather aggregated level, the interrelationship between life style, environment, human biology, the health services, and health status. From a provincial point of view, which is where health planning has its reality, the results of the Canada Health Survey will resemble an atlas whereas what is more appropriate at this level is a scale of 1/508,880[5] — a sample designed less to give an account of *all* the health fields than a detailed picture of the single most important objective of the health services about which we have next to no information – ill health. An information base of this kind is implied by each of the Mustard task force's nine specific responsibilities for district health councils. In particular, three of them identify it quite specifically.

(3) Planning for the district in a co-ordinated spectrum of programs in the primary and secondary care sectors and planning the development of both public and private facilities. This would involve establishing objectives, identifying needs, evaluating alternatives and establishing priorities as to how existing needs could best be met to ensure the most effective use of resources ... (5) Ensuring that methods exist in the district for effective and appropriate evaluation of health services and that suitable arrangements exist for taking corrective action when required. This would include ensuring that quality of care was maintained

5 This happens to be the scale (8 miles to 1 inch) of map no. 33A Ontario Electoral Districts.

and that effective mechanisms were established for internal and external audit of health services and for internal and external peer review of health professionals ... (9) Establishing an effective information system to supply data on community needs and to draw on health services information compiled at the Ministry level. The Council must have access to such information as it needs to carry out its functions. (Task Force, 1974, 25-7)

It should be noted moreover, that even the data generated by a detailed community-based survey could never be sufficient for adequate monitoring of institutions, or for use in peer review. If the appropriate base for evaluating community needs both now and in the future must be the community itself, and not health institutions, so one appropriate base for monitoring the performance of institutions must be the institutions – or rather the patients they serve. We say '*one* appropriate base' for the evaluation of institutions such as primary care units or hospitals because, while quality of care, etc., given to patients treated in health care organizations is an important dimension of the effectiveness of their functioning, it should *never* be the only base. While physicians have generally regarded their responsibility as being towards *their own patients*, an efficient *system* must be evaluated in terms of its impact upon *all* patients and upon *the health of those who may never actually become patients*. The community, then, is not merely the right base for evaluating needs but also one of the bases for evaluating the effectiveness of local institutions which serve these needs. Even if it may be regarded as proper for the individual physician to see his duty only in terms of providing the best service he can for his own patients, irrespective of the resources he draws away from other doctors' patients or from potential patients not in touch with the system – and the properness of this might, of course, be reasonably questioned – it cannot be regarded as either proper or – what is the same thing – conducive to the better health of the whole community for the *system* to be monitored and evaluated on this basis. Thus, even if the physician can see his duty as beginning only with the first consultation, the community cannot.

RESEARCH PRIORITIES

The latter part of the previous section also leads us naturally into a discussion of the uses of health measures as priority indicators in other matters than geographical. For the sake of illustration we shall here focus on just one of the types mentioned in the introductory part of the present chapter: medical and medical care research.

The problem of deciding priorities in health research in Ontario has recently been reviewed and discussed by Fraser (1972). It is not our purpose here to travel this route again but to show how health measures may aid in the decisions confronting those whose responsibility is to fund medical and related research.

As with other attempts to derive criteria for research funding we shall have little to say about what is commonly called 'basic' research but rather concentrate on those kinds of research commonly referred to as 'applied' and 'developmental' (for a full discussion of these and other classifications of health research, see Fraser (1972, part I).

The kind of criteria developed by Fraser are either rather crude guides based upon disease-specific mortality or much more sophisticated calculations of potential 'benefit' from disease-specific programs based upon the kind of 'benefit' calculation commonly made in cost-benefit analyses. Unfortunately, even the more sophisticated of these attempts (e.g., Weisbrod, 1971) resemble far more the financial investment appraisal criteria used in industry than the social cost-benefit criteria that are appropriate if the arguments in chapters two and three of this work are accepted. Not only do they tend to place an undue emphasis on mortality but value life-years gained according to the contribution of those lives to the national (provincial) income – the maximization of which is not, we have supposed, the objective of the provincial health services. Ultimately, of course, it is true that the potential benefits of a research project must be weighed against its expected costs and this process does inescapably involve (at the least) an *implicit* valuation of the benefits in monetary terms. In our view, however, to focus on the inherent difficulties of this dollar valuation process, or, alternatively to rush into it with a determined looking GPP orientation, quite apart from the substantial antagonism it frequently, and not altogether unjustifiably, generates in the medical profession, is a tactical error that holds back the rational development and appraisal of research programs, as well as leaving far too much in the quantitative field in the hands of the philistines – or at least those who will find only philistine uses for the data by assuming, for example, that what is numerical and dollar-valued must be larger than what is (currently) non-numerical and qualitative.

A much more important problem, which is logically prior to the valuation problem, concerns the measurement of unexpected outcomes not merely in terms of the impact on mortality, but in terms of impact on the state of health of the entire client population whether defined by disease, social class, race, sex, or geographical characteristics (of these, a disease grouping implies research primarily into the causes and the management of disease while the others are concerned with the effective delivery of care with epidemiological work embracing all aspects).

The contribution made by a particular disease to an index of community ill-health is, of course, a measure (embodying values though not money prices) that is an estimate of the gains in health available as the result of the application of new medical knowledge or procedures. It would seem highly desirable for potential researchers to display an awareness of the productivity of their work, if successful, and they should be both encouraged to formulate proposals bearing this in mind and be evaluated by sponsors in turn using this as one of their criteria. Indeed, so far as the *productivity* of research is concerned, its impact on ability to function in a pain and anxiety free way, and the associated changes in treatment, etc., cost is a necessary criterion. The other relevant criteria for evaluating research are, of course, its cost and the probability of its success (of which the competence of the researchers themselves is an important indicator).

Fraser (1972) presents an excellent summary of the present state of (economic) thinking about health research. Particularly noticeable in this genre is the emphasis, as we have pointed out above, on financial variables — particularly the potential savings from prevention programs (see especially Fraser, 1972, part V). This emphasis leads Fraser to place among the '*indirect* costs of ill-health' (p.22 ff.) the pain and suffering of disease, which are held to be very difficult to measure. As Karman (1965, 100) has observed: 'A pervasive problem in economic calculations is the tendency to measure and report what is readily measurable; and that is not necessarily relevant or most important. The less tangible losses, such as pain and grief, are not measured. This is tantamount to valuing them at zero.'

This 'indirect' cost of disease is, of course, precisely what the Wolfson health indexes discussed above attempt to measure. Insofar as the strength of aversion to a particular disease would include views about lack of functioning, pain, and distress, and a view of likely duration (as is presumable the case with the Wolfson index) it is possible to claim for it quite an (implicitly) all-embracing nature, though that nature does not include the differential income-consequences that may exist in diseases having a different incidence in different socio-economic classes, or different age-groups.

Table 17 presents a list of those diseases that were sufficiently serious to warrant admission to hospital in 1974. Columns (*a*) and (*c*) show the total numbers of separations unweighted and weighted by the Wolfson HHI index respectively. Columns (*b*), (*d*), and (*e*) show into which of ten ranked classes each disease fell when measured by separations, weighted separations, and the Wolfson weights respectively. The ten classes (shown at the bottom of the table) each include roughly 20 diseases, with the exception of the highest ranked class containing rather fewer 'major' diseases and the tenth, which contains a larger number of diseases of either low incidence, small importance, or both.

TABLE 17

Separations from Ontario active general rehabilitations and special rehabilitation hospitals in 1974, weighted by severity index of primary diagnosis (excluding mental disorders)

Ontario broad code list of 260 diagnostic categories (2) ICDA-8 Ontario section broad code	Total separations (a)	Rank class no. of separations (b)	Separations weighted by severity (c)	Rank class by weighted separations (d)	Rank class by severity of one case of the disease (e)
I *Infective and parasitic diseases*					
001 Salmonella infections, cholera, and typhoid	239	10	0.84	10	9
002 Gastroenteritis and colitis, food poisoning, specified intestinal infection	18,805	1	50.77	4	9
003 Diarrhea	1657	7	4.47	9	9
004 Tuberculosis	867	9	39.45	5	5
005 Zoonosis	21	10	0.21	10	7
006 Whooping cough, specified and unspecified bacterial diseases	916	9	18.32	7	6
007 Streptococcal sore throat, scarlet fever and erysipelas	475	10	0.48	10	10
008 Meningococcal infection and tetanus	120	10	30.00	5	2
009 Septicemia	550	9	45.87	5	4
010 Poliomyelitis	8	10	0.81	10	3
011 Acute poliomyelitis unspecified	17	10	1.75	10	3
012 Late effects of acute poliomyelitis	75	10	0.52	10	8
013 Aseptic meningitis, specified enterovirus diseases of central nervous system	310	10	1.86	10	8
014 Viral diseases accompanied by exanthem	1800	7	7.20	9	9
015 Arthroped borne viral diseases	163	10	1.04	10	8
016 Viral diseases—warts, infections, mononucleosis, mumps, specified and unspecified diseases	4401	5	4.40	9	10

017	Infectious hepatitis	965	9	15.54	7	6
018	Venereal diseases	1039	8	1.04	10	10
019	Vincents angina, malaria, specified and unspecified spirochetal diseases	129	10	0.77	10	8
020	Sarcoidosis, moniliasis, pinworms, specified and unspecified infective and parasitic diseases	1147	8	4.59	9	9
II	*Neoplasms*					
021	Malignant neoplasm of buccal cavity and pharynx	1288	8	19.32	7	6
022	Malignant neoplasm of stomach	1702	7	1055.24	2	1
023	Malignant neoplasm of small intestine including duodenum	75	10	47.25	5	1
024	Malignant neoplasm of large intestine except rectum	4019	5	1004.75	2	2
025	Malignant neoplasm of rectum and rectosigmoid junction	2020	7	606.00	2	2
026	Malignant neoplasm of pancreas, specified and unspecified digestive organs	2198	7	1758.40	1	1
027	Malignant neoplasm of trachea	21	10	15.33	7	1
028	Malignant neoplasm of bronchus and lung	6519	3	4758.87	1	1
029	Malignant neoplasm of larynx, nose, specified and unspecified respiratory organs	939	9	685.47	2	1
030	Malignant neoplasm of bone	646	9	503.88	2	1
031	Malignant neoplasm of skin	1819	7	32.74	5	6
032	Malignant neoplasm of breast	6750	3	2025.00	1	2
033	Malignant neoplasm of cervix uteri	2004	7	501.00	2	2
034	Malignant neoplasm of uterus	1614	7	645.60	2	2
035	Malignant neoplasm of ovary	1324	8	529.00	2	2
036	Malignant neoplasm of fallopian tube and broad ligament	74	10	29.60	2	2

TABLE 17, *continued*

Separations from Ontario active general rehabilitations and special rehabilitation hospitals in 1974, weighted by severity index of primary diagnosis (excluding mental disorders)

Ontario broad code list of 260 diagnostic categories (2) / ICDA-8 Ontario section broad code	Total separations (a)	Rank class no. of separations (b)	Separations weighted by severity (c)	Rank class by weighted separations (d)	Rank class by severity of one case of the disease (e)
037 Malignant neoplasm of vulva, specified female genital organs	310	10	55.8	4	3
038 Malignant neoplasm of prostate	3413	6	621.17	2	3
039 Malignant neoplasm of testes, specified male genital organs	372	10	74.20	4	2
040 Malignant neoplasm of bladder	3202	6	960.60	2	2
041 Malignant neoplasm of kidney, specified urinary organs	833	9	416.50	2	2
042 Malignant neoplasm of brain	478	10	430.20	2	1
043 Malignant neoplasms, primary and secondary specified parts of nervous system, thyroid gland, multiple sites, ill-defined sites	6109	3	2443.60	1	2
044 Leukemia	3057	6	2353.89	1	1
045 Hodgkins disease, lymphosarcoma, multiple myeloma, specified neoplasms-lymphatic and hematopoietic tissue	5372	4	1611.60	1	2
046 Benign neoplasm of breast	2170	7	1.74	10	10
047 Benign neoplasm of skin	385	10	0.04	10	10
048 Benign neoplasm of uterus	10,269	2	25.67	6	9
049 Benign neoplasm of ovary	3757	5	9.39	8	9
050 Benign neoplasm of vulva, specified female genital organs	1085	8	2.71	10	9
051 Benign neoplasm of male genital organs	25	10	0.01	10	10

No.					
052 Benign neoplasm—peripheral nerves, brain specified parts of nervous system	682	9	17.05	7	5
053 Benign neoplasm—exostosis, hemangioma, lipoma, rectum, large intestine specified and unspecified sites	6715	3	21.49	6	9
054 Carcinoma in situ of cervix uteri	1607	7	32.14	5	6
055 Unspecified neoplasm—breast, bladder, brain specified and unspecified sites	4057	5	81.14	4	6
III *Endocrine, nutritional and metabolic diseases*					
056 Thyrotoxicosis with or without goiter	909	9	14.54	8	6
057 Nontoxic goiter	1265	8	2.53	10	10
058 Myxidema, specified and unspecified disease of thyroid gland	890	9	17.80	7	6
059 Diabetes mellitus	16,806	1	862.15	2	4
060 Disorder of pancreatic secretion, ovarian dysfunction, adrenal cortical hypofunction, specified and unspecified endocrine diseases	2066	7	51.65	4	5
061 Nutritional marasmus	43	10	4.30	9	3
062 Nutritional and vitamin deficiencies, malabsorption syndrome, sprue	2294	7	11.47	8	8
063 Congenital disorders of metabolism	869	9	139.04	3	3
064 Obesity, gout, specified and unspecified metabolic diseases	2160	7	97.20	4	5
IV *Diseases of the blood and blood-forming organs*					
065 Iron deficiency anemias	1318	8	3.82	10	9
066 Pernicious, folic acid, specified and unspecified deficiency anemias	604	9	2.42	10	9
067 Mesenteric lymphadenitis, anemia thrombocytopenia, specified diseases of blood and blood-forming organs	7391	3	1108.65	2	3

TABLE 17, *continued*

Separations from Ontario active general rehabilitations and special rehabilitation hospitals in 1974, weighted by severity index of primary diagnosis (excluding mental disorders)

Ontario broad code list of 260 diagnostic categories (2) ICDA-8 Ontario section broad code	Total separations (a)	Rank class no. of separations (b)	Separations weighted by severity (c)	Rank class by weighted separations (d)	Rank class by severity of one case of the disease (e)
VI *Diseases of the nervous system and sense organs*					
077 Meningitis, encephalitis, myelitis, specified diseases of central nervous system	1023	8	102.30	3	3
078 Hereditary diseases—neuromuscular disorders, diseases of the striatopallidal system, ataxia	352	10	225.28	3	1
079 Other specified and unspecified hereditary and familial diseases of nervous system	22	10	15.40	7	1
080 Multiple sclerosis	1129	8	486.71	2	2
081 Paralysis agitans	1055	8	63.30	4	4
082 Epilepsy	3841	5	65.68	4	6
083 Migraine, cerebral atrophy, specified and unspecified brain and motor neurone disease	3118	6	28.06	6	7
084 Menoplegia, paraplegia, specified and unspecified diseases of central nervous system	2924	6	438.60	2	3
085 Diseases of nerves and peripheral ganglia	5813	4	34.88	5	8
086 Conjunctivitis and ophthalmia	204	10	0.04	10	10
087 Inflammatory diseases of the eye	1642	7	1.64	10	10
088 Strabismus	4784	4	7.18	9	10
089 Cataract	10,897	2	49.04	5	9
090 Glaucoma	1306	8	6.53	9	8

No.	Disease				
091	Detachment of retina, blepharochalasis specified and unspecified diseases of the eye	4118	5	4.12	9	10
092	Otitis media without mention of mastoiditis	9098	2	7.28	9	10
093	Mastoiditis with or without otitis media	716	9	7.16	9	7
094	Otosclerosis, perforation of tympanic membrane, labyrinthitis, specified and unspecified diseases of ear and mastoid process	4688	4	14.06	8	9

VII *Diseases of the circulatory system*

No.	Disease				
095	Active rheumatic fever	377	10	5.66	9	6
096	Chronic rheumatic heart disease	3391	6	558.50	2	3
097	Hypertensive disease	8469	2	552.18	2	4
098	Acute myocardial infarction	19,303	1	3474.54	1	3
099	Ischemic heart disease—chronic acute, coronary insufficiency, angina pectoris, others specified	39,562	1	7121.16	1	3
100	Congestive heart failure, atrial fibrillation, heart block, specified unspecified forms of heart disease	18,846	1	5653.80	1	2
101	Cerebral hemorrhage	1098	8	215.21	3	3
102	Cerebral embolism and thrombosis	3598	5	719.60	2	2
103	Cerebrovascular disease—acute, ischemic, transient	15,615	1	6246.00	1	2
104	Arteriosclerosis	2468	7	160.42	3	4
105	Aortic aneurysm	1194	8	298.50	3	2
106	Peripheral vascular disease, gangrene, embolism and thrombosis, aneurysm specified and unspecified diseases of arteries, arterioles and capillaries	6853	3	822.36	2	3
107	Pulmonary embolism and infarction	2396	7	479.20	2	2
108	Phlebitis and thrombophlebitis	4025	5	120.75	3	5
109	Venous embolism and thrombosis	981	9	98.10	4	3

TABLE 17, continued

Separations from Ontario active general rehabilitations and special rehabilitation hospitals in 1974, weighted by severity index of primary diagnosis (excluding mental disorders)

Ontario broad code list of 260 diagnostic categories (2) ICDA-8 Ontario section broad code	Total separations (a)	Rank class no. of separations (b)	Separations weighted by severity (c)	Rank class by weighted separations (d)	Rank class by severity of one case of the disease (e)
VII *Diseases of the circulatory system*					
110 Varicose veins of lower extremities	9047	2	28.95	6	9
111 Hemorrhoids	7545	3	18.11	7	9
112 Non-infective disease of lymphatic channels	187	10	1.50	10	7
113 Varix-esophagus, scrotum, specified and unspecified diseases of circulatory system	1508	7	15.08	7	7
VII *Diseases of the respiratory system*					
114 Acute upper respiratory infection except influenza	30,068	1	9.02	8	10
115 Influenza	2758	6	1.38	10	10
116 Pneumonia	22,958	1	126.27	3	8
117 Bronchitis	12,394	2	12.39	8	10
118 Emphysema	2196	7	185.34	3	4
119 Asthma	11,967	2	434.40	2	5
120 Hypertrophy of tonsils and adenoids	51,579	1	10.32	8	10
121 Chronic sinusitis	1756	7	11.06	8	8
122 Deflected nasal septum	7299	3	1.46	10	10
123 Polyps of nose, vocal cords, larynx specified and unspecified diseases of the upper respiratory tract	5675	4	5.11	9	10
124 Empyema and abscess of lung	262	10	18.34	7	4

125	Pneumoconiosis and related diseases	95	10	11.40	8	3
126	Pulmonary congestion, spontaneous pneumothorax, pleurisy, specified diseases of respiratory system	3357	6	33.57	5	7
127	Chronic interstitial pneumonia, bronchiectasis, specified and unspecified lung diseases	6610	3	264.40	3	5
IX	*Diseases of the digestive system*					
128	Diseases of teeth and supporting structures	22,928	1	16.05	7	10
129	Stomatitis, sialothiasis, specified diseases of jaws and oral soft tissues	1793	7	3.59	10	10
130	Diseases of esophagus	2392	7	23.92	6	7
131	Ulcer of stomach	3212	6	80.94	4	5
132	Ulcer of duodenum	9297	2	234.29	3	5
133	Peptic ulcer, site unspecified	1858	7	46.82	5	5
134	Gastrojejunal ulcer	108	10	3.24	10	5
135	Gastritis and duodenitis	5728	4	11.46	8	10
136	Gastrointestinal disorder, pyloric stenosis acquired, specified and unspecified diseases of stomach and duodenum	1397	8	13.97	8	7
137	Appendicitis	15,477	1	37.14	5	9
138	Hernia without mention of obstruction	33,329	1	189.98	3	8
139	Hernia with obstruction	1280	8	25.60	6	6
140	Intestinal obstruction without mention of hernia	4621	4	138.63	3	5
141	Gastroenteritis and colitis, except ulcerative, of non-infectious origin	57	10	0.17	10	9
142	Chronic enteritis and ulcerative colitis	2260	7	101.70	3	5
143	Diverticula of intestine	4807	4	48.07	5	7

TABLE 17, *continued*

Separations from Ontario active general rehabilitations and special rehabilitation hospitals in 1974, weighted by severity index of primary diagnosis (excluding mental disorders)

Ontario broad code list of 260 diagnostic categories (2) / ICDA-8 Ontario section broad code	Total separations (*a*)	Rank class no of separations (*b*)	Separations weighted by severity (*c*)	Rank class by weighted separations (*d*)	Rank class by severity of one case of the disease (*e*)
IX *Diseases of the digestive system*					
144 Anal fissure, anal fistula, anal abscess, constipation, specified diseases of intestines and peritoneum	12,662	2	151.14	3	7
145 Cirrhosis of liver	4969	4	2653.45	1	2
146 Hepatitis, specified and unspecified diseases of liver	1133	8	679.80	2	1
147 Cholelithiasis	25,733	1	66.91	4	9
148 Cholecystitis and cholangitis, without mention of calculus	8303	2	41.51	5	8
149 Obstruction, specified and unspecified diseases of gallbladder and biliary ducts	1055	8	21.10	6	6
150 Diseases of pancreas	3032	6	151.60	3	4
X *Diseases of the genito-urinary system*					
151 Nephritis and nephrosis	27,035	1	4055.25	1	3
152 Infections of kidney	4085	5	81.70	4	6
153 Hydronephrosis	729	9	68.96	4	4
154 Calculus of urinary system	9393	2	140.90	3	6
155 Cystitis	4076	5	26.09	6	8
156 Contracture of bladder sphincter specified and unspecified diseases of bladder	1595	7	31.90	5	6

X   *Diseases of the genito-urinary system*

157	Stricture of urethra	3828	5	70.44	4	6
158	Urinary tract infection, renal disease, urethritis, specified and unspecified diseases of urinary system	9406	2	112.87	3	7
159	Hyperplasia of prostate	9676	2	17.42	7	10
160	Redundant prepuse and phimosis	3489	6	0.70	10	10
161	Hydrocele, prostatitis, epididymitis, specified diseases of male genital organs	5737	4	22.95	6	9
162	Diseases of breast	6477	3	6.48	9	10
163	Diseases of ovary, fallopian tube and parametrium	7115	3	14.23	8	10
164	Infective diseases of cervix uteri	4367	5	6.55	9	10
165	Infective diseases of uterus except cervix, vagina, and vulva	2090	7	4.18	9	10
166	Uterovaginal prolapse	9263	2	59.28	4	8
167	Malposition of uterus	715	9	0.21	10	10
168	Disorders of menstruation	25,655	1	76.97	4	9
169	Endometriosis, sterility hyperplasia of endometrium, specified and unspecified diseases of uterus and female genital organs	11,072	2	77.50	4	8

XI   *Complications of pregnancy, childbirth and the puerperium*

170	Infections of genital tract during pregnancy and urinary infections during pregnancy and puerperium	928	9	7.42	9	7
171	Hemorrhage of pregnancy	5201	4	281.37	3	4
172	False labour, ectopic pregnancy, missed abortion, specified and unspecified complications of pregnancy	17,961	1	53.90	4	9

TABLE 17, *continued*

Separations from Ontario active general rehabilitations and special rehabilitation hospitals in 1974, weighted by severity index of primary diagnosis (excluding mental disorders)

Ontario broad code list of 260 diagnostic categories (2) ICDA-8 Ontario section broad code	Total separations (a)	Rank class no of separations (b)	Separations weighted by severity (c)	Rank class by weighted separations (d)	Rank class by severity of one case of the disease (e)
XI *Complications of pregnancy, childbirth and the puerperium*					
173 Pre-eclampsia, eclampsia, toxemia unspecified and hyperemesis gravidarum	3268	6	130.72	3	5
174 Renal disease, specified toxemias of pregnancy and the puerperium	53	10	2.65	10	4
175 Abortion	30,468	1	15.23	7	10
177 Delivery complicated by—placenta previa or antepartum hemorrhage, retained placenta or other postpartum hemorrhage	2711	6	94.89	4	5
178 Delivery complicated by bony pelvis	79	10	0.28	10	9
179 Delivery complicated by fetopelvic disproportion	3236	6	11.33	8	9
180 Delivery complicated by malpresentation of fetus	2685	6	32.22	5	7
181 Delivery complicated by prolonged labour of other origin	1922	7	4.81	9	9
182 Delivery with laceration of perineum, previous cesarean section, specified and unspecified complications	17,380	1	52.14	4	9
183 Complications of puerperium	1530	7	9.18	8	8

XII *Diseases of the skin and subcutaneous tissue*

184	Impetigo	300	10	0.03	10	10
185	Pilonidal cyst	3325	6	1.66	10	10
186	Infections of skin and subcutaneous tissue	5411	4	1.08	10	10
187	Eczema, dermatitis, psoriasis, specified and unspecified inflammatory conditions of skin and subcutaneous tissue	4468	5	1.34	10	10
188	Ingrowing nail, cicatrix, sebaceous cyst, skin ulcer, specified and unspecified diseases of skin and subcutaneous tissue	8195	2	2.46	10	10

XIII *Diseases of musculoskeletal system and connective tissue*

189	Rheumatoid arthritis and allied conditions	4736	4	395.46	2	4
190	Osteoarthritis and allied conditions	7066	3	113.06	3	6
191	Specified and unspecified arthritis and rheumatism	4857	4	26.71	6	8
192	Osteomyelitis, osteoporosis, juvenile osteochondrosis of hip, specified diseases of bone	3993	5	71.87	4	6
193	Displacement of intervertebral disc	15,703	1	284.22	3	6
194	Knee derangement, joint dislocations, lumbalgia, specified and unspecified disease of joints	14,974	2	89.84	4	8
195	Synovitis, bursitis and tenosynovitis	6076	3	24.30	6	9
196	Hallux valgus, deformity of toe, contracture of palmar fascia, specified and unspecified diseases of musculoskeletal system	9139	2	73.11	4	7

TABLE 17, *continued*

Separations from Ontario active general rehabilitations and special rehabilitation hospitals in 1974, weighted by severity index of primary diagnosis (excluding mental disorders)

Ontario broad code list of 260 diagnostic categories (2) / ICDA-8 Ontario section broad code	Total separations (a)	Rank class no of separations (b)	Separations weighted by severity (c)	Rank class by weighted separations (d)	Rank class by severity of one case of the disease (e)
XIV *Congenital anomalies*					
197 Spina bifida and congenital hydrocephalus	584	9	146.00	3	2
198 Neurofibromatosis, specified and unspecified congenital anomalies of nervous system	242	10	60.50	4	2
199 Congenital anomalies of eye	280	10	1.26	10	9
200 Anomalies of ear	927	9	9.27	8	7
201 Congenital anomalies of heart	1897	7	18.97	7	3
202 Patent ductus arteriosus, coarctation of aorta and other anomalies of aorta	350	10	26.25	6	4
203 Stenosis of pulmonary artery, specified and unspecified congenital anomalies of circulatory system	269	10	20.18	6	4
204 Specified and unspecified congenital anomalies of nose	51	10	0.51	10	7
205 Cleft palate	241	10	2.41	10	7
206 Cleft lip	240	10	2.40	10	7
207 Cleft palate with cleft lip	160	10	1.60	10	7
208 Pyloric stenosis, congenital meckels diverticulum, specified and unspecified congenital anomalies of digestive system	1182	8	29.55	6	5
209 Congenital anomalies of genito-urinary system	3084	6	15.42	7	8

210	Clubfoot–congenital	749	9	11.83	8	6
211	Congenital anomalies of musculoskeletal system	2577	6	77.31	4	5
212	Anomalies–skin, thyroid gland, Down's disease, specified and unspecified congenital anomalies	1792	7	17.92	7	7
XV	*Certain causes of perinatal morbidity and mortality*					
213	Chronic circulatory and genito-urinary diseases in mother	2	10	0.20	10	3
214	Diabetes, specified and unspecified maternal conditions unrelated to pregnancy	13	10	0.59	10	5
215	Toxemia of pregnancy	5	10	0.29	10	5
216	Maternal ante- and intrapartum infection	1	10	0.01	10	7
217	Birth injury	67	10	3.01	10	5
218	Asphyxia, anoxia, or hypoxia	838	9	37.71	5	5
219	Hemolytic disease of newborn	161	10	17.23	7	3
220	Immaturity unspecified–excludes immature newborn	213	10	14.91	8	4
221	Hemorrhagic disease of newborn	15	10	0.68	10	5
222	Newborn–physiological jaundice, umbilical cord conditions, specified and unspecified diseases and conditions	686	9	30.87	5	5
223	Termination of pregnancy	1	10	0.00	10	10
XVII	*Accidents, poisonings and violence – nature of injury*					
226	Fracture of skull	558	9	5.58	9	7
227	Fracture of jaw	2068	7	15.51	7	7

TABLE 17, *continued*

Separations from Ontario active general rehabilitations and special rehabilitation hospitals in 1974, weighted by severity index of primary diagnosis (excluding mental disorders)

Ontario broad code list of 260 diagnostic categories (2) ICDA-8 Ontario section broad code	Total separations (a)	Rank class no of separations (b)	Separations weighted by severity (c)	Rank class by weighted separations (d)	Rank class by severity of one case of the disease (e)
XVII *Accidents, poisonings and violence – nature of injury (continued)*					
228 Fracture – skull and face bones, multiple and late effects	4356	5	32.67	5	7
229 Fractures of spine and trunk	7403	3	111.04	3	6
230 Fracture of upper limb	11,675	2	35.02	5	9
231 Fracture of femur	9734	2	146.01	3	6
232 Fracture – tibia, fibula, patella, sites of lower limbs	11,390	2	45.56	5	9
233 Dislocation without fracture, sprains of joints and adjacent muscles	7450	3	7.45	9	10
234 Intracranial injury excluding those with skull fracture	16,477	1	197.72	3	7
235 Intracranial injury without mention of open intracranial wound	752	9	112.80	3	3
236 Intracranial injury with open intracranial wound	6	10	0.90	10	3
237 Intracranial injury – late effects	13	10	1.95	10	3
238 Internal injury of chest, abdomen and pelvis	2445	7	183.38	3	4
239 Head, neck and trunk – laceration, multiple wounds, without complication, complicated, late effects	2147	7	4.29	9	10

240	Open wound of eye and ear	690	9	48.64	5	4
241	Traumatic amputation of upper limbs	955	9	28.65	6	5
242	Traumatic amputation of lower limbs	182	10	9.10	8	4
243	Limbs and unspecified sites – open and multiple wounds, superficial injury, without complication, complicated, late effects	7050	3	14.10	8	10
244	Contusion and crushing with intact skin surfaces	5494	4	0.55	10	10
245	Effects of foreign body entering through orifice	1688	7	0.84	10	10
246	Burns	3578	5	17.89	7	8
247	Injury to nerves and spinal cord	1191	8	59.55	4	4
248	Adverse effects of medical agents	12,044	2	301.10	2	5
249	Toxic effects of substances chiefly non-medicinal as to source	1892	7	45.41	5	6
250	Injury unspecified – trunk, knee and unspecified sites, frostbite and specified adverse effects	3518	5	14.07	8	9
251	Complication peculiar to certain surgical and medical procedures	9013	2	360.52	2	5

TABLE 17, *continued*

Separations from Ontario active general rehabilitations and special rehabilitation hospitals in 1974, weighted by severity index of primary diagnosis (excluding mental disorders)

Rank class	(b) Separations	(d) Weighted separations	(e) Wolfson weights
1	>15,000	>1500	>0.5999
2	8000–15,000	300–1500.00	0.2 –0.5999
3	6000– 7900	100– 299.99	0.1 –0.1999
4	4500– 8999	50– 99.99	0.05 –0.0999
5	3500– 4499	30– 49.99	0.025 –0.0499
6	2500– 3499	20– 29.99	0.015 –0.0249
7	1500– 2499	15– 19.99	0.0075–0.0149
8	1000– 1499	9– 14.99	0.005 –0.0074
9	500– 999	4– 8.99	0.0024–0.0049
10	>500	>4	>0.0024

SOURCES: Wolfson (1974); Ontario Ministry of Health (*Hospital Statistics 1974*, Table 13)
NOTES: The rank classes corresponding to columns (*b*), (*d*), and (*e*) are listed above.

It is immediately clear that the ranking of diseases according to the demand they make on hospital space[6] is not the same as that according to their intrinsic undesirability (see, e.g., code nos. 002, 092, 128). Conversely, diseases having a relatively low incidence can rise to the highest priority categories: 146, 105. Some evidence of the validity of an index of this sort is given by the fact that the cancers, heart disease, and other old favourites come out high which seems in accordance with common concern. Such diseases, however, which strike mainly at older persons, tend to have lower priority in the financial indexes for the simple reason that such persons have few, if any, remaining working days.

It is thus our claim that indexes of this sort add a valuable new element into the calculus of research and may refute the tendency to support that what cannot (or could not) be measured must be either unimportant or small. It would, of course, be wrong to suppose that index (c) measures *all* one wishes to know about the benefit side of treatment or research. Obviously, for practical purposes, the basis for the calculations in Table 17 is far too restricted. But emphasis on the financial gain from rapid cure or prevention per dollar spent ought at the least to be set alongside estimates of the reduction in the total index of ill-health per dollar spent. If we cannot instruct the decision-maker how he should trade these two off, at least we can help him quantify that which he will have to trade off. As the pressures mount upon the government to control public expenditure on health care, including subtle areas like research, it is surely important that the quantification of potential outcomes does not stop with financial considerations. As Somers and Somers say, 'the satisfactions purchased in health care are not exclusively, probably not even primarily, economic. There are humanitarian values, religious values respecting human life, social values and personal values such as sheer comfort and relief from pain and anxiety' (1967, p. 27). If for 'economic' we read 'financial' (which is what is surely meant, regrettable though this vulgar identification is) then this quotation puts us precisely on guard against a new philistinism, which health status indexes help us quantitatively to combat.

MONITORING PERFORMANCE AND QUALITY OF CARE

Although it has become common, following Donabedian (1966), to distinguish evaluation of *structure* (physical resources, organizational frame, qualifications of personnel) from evaluation of *process* (care supplied as judged by given norms) and from evaluation of *outcomes* or *output* (effect on health status), we view the former as essentially *contributory* to the third which is the ultimate, and ultimately the only, criterion by which the former should be evaluated.

---

6 Separations are, of course, only a very rough guide to the costliness of the disease since no allowance is made for length of stay, case complexity, etc.

The dangers of focusing on the former as proxies for the latter have been often identified (e.g., Brook, 1973b). The major one is an obsession with 'what goes in' rather than 'what comes out' – not all are as liberated from an input orientation as A.L. Cochrane, who has compared hospitals with crematoria ('so much goes in and so little comes out') (Cochrane, 1975, 282). Regardless of the accuracy of his observation, the striking analogy makes a good point: what goes in can be evaluated only in terms of what comes out. Unfortunately, the temptation for everyone to slip into the mistake of evaluating quality without reference to 'what comes out' is made harder to resist since virtually every piece of statistical information relating to primary or secondary care relates to inputs. The assumption is well-nigh universal that *more* (more resources, more qualifications, more everything) means better care.

The recent report *Evaluation of Primary Health Care Services* in Ontario (Ontario Council of Health, 1976) is refreshingly aware of this distinction but, aside from a hope that the Canada Health Survey may yield some useful data, has no really strong (or new) points to make. Most of its recommendations relate to structure and process. Examination of process is a good deal better than emphasis on structure, since it encourages good record keeping and enables identification of *prima facie* cases of incompetence or error (e.g., wrong diagnosis and/or treatment given unambiguous symptoms) and encourages the adoption of effective techniques and aids to better diagnosis and treatment as seem, for example, now possible by the use of computers (e.g., de Dombal *et al.*, 1972) and the use of randomized controlled trials (where feasible) to test clinical effectiveness. But even better would be an emphasis, at the level of individual hospitals and individual physicians, on outcome in the sense of the *difference* their efforts make to patients' ability to function in society without pain, stress, etc. (that is, the difference in patients' health status, both actual and prospective, before and after). A view that is very close to the emphasis on prognostic outcome by Williamson (1971). A further deficiency of process criteria – and even of outcome and accessibility criteria as proposed by the Ontario Council of Health – is that performance is evaluated in terms of *persons processed* rather than *community served*. This deficiency is inherent in an *institutional* view of the issues and while it is a worthy aim to seek to identify (for example) patient satisfaction and patient convenience (as regards distance from a unit, car parking facilities, etc.) this is *not* measurement of the quality of care from the community viewpoint, which has to relate to the *community* and not merely to patients. The person who found accessibility so difficult that he did not actually turn up will not get counted at all.

Even in the evaluation of institutions then, we are compelled to look beyond the institutions themselves and the clients they actually serve, and for this there can be no substitute for a community-based survey of functional ability which would, of course, include patients actually cared for. But even within an institutional frame that did focus only on process, or persons processed, there remains much to be done.

There is an understandable reluctance to use some of the existing data that could quite readily be obtained, such as case-fatality rates for individual hospital physicians. Its source would seem to be three-fold: (*a*) the stress their use would impose upon the individual doctors; (*b*) the misinterpretations that would be possible; (*c*) the counter-productive incentives their use may provide. We propose here to discuss only (*b*) and (*c*) on the grounds that aside from these causes, there should be no additional stress for the conscientious physician who was not ashamed to have his work monitored by his peers.

Although there have been studies using explicit outcome measures such as case-fatality rates for hospitals (for an early example, see Lipworth *et al.*, 1963) such data, whether for institutions or individual practitioners, are determined by many factors other than those deriving from personal skills: the severity of presenting symptoms, ages of patients, facilities, and resources available to the doctor, etc. In addition, it is quite unreasonable to expect the average physician's skills to be as good as those of the very best. Such considerations should not, however, lead us to reject on *a priori* grounds an attempt to monitor clinical effectiveness but rather to experiment with available data to see, for example, whether those whose ostensible output was (say) two standard deviations below average turned out upon more detailed peer review to have unacceptably low levels of competence. Similarly, they should not discourage an attempt to devise simple indicators of functioning at least for those procedures (orthopedics?) where outcome could be fairly readily assessed in terms of physical mobility.

The Ontario Council of Health (1976, 5) 'recognized the importance of outcome indicators and measurement, but because of time constraints and methodological problems, did not include these as a separate activity.' This was unfortunate for, so long as we do not let the perfect become the enemy of the merely good, there is much scope for their use, even if they are crude. Even relatively 'quick and dirty' indicators have, judiciously interpreted, a promise which should be tested experimentally.

The dangers of false incentives would clearly apply if even sophisticated instruments were used naively and *a fortiori* with cruder measures. An awareness of the methodology expounded in chapters four and five, however, would temper their immoderate use which should remain mainly that of identifying *prima facie* poor practice for subsequent more detailed peer review. It is manifestly of central importance that clinicians not be encouraged by any monitoring system to be *unduly* risk-averse.

It is worth noting that monitoring *process* is not without its adverse disincentive effects. The rise of malpractice suits in the USA, for example, has (it is often alleged) led to physicians not only refraining from using procedures which may cure the patient but which have a higher risk of failure and exposure to the threat of a lawsuit, but also, as protection against lawsuits, to engage in excessive pathology, X-ray, etc., tests which normally would not be required. One may also suspect that by encouraging the non-treatment of 'risky' cases some such patients have effectively been 'turned away' from the system.

Thus, even quality of care evaluation, especially when at the level of an entire institution such as a primary care unit or a hospital, cannot escape — always supposing the idea is really to be taken seriously — a community basis of approach. Nor will all the monitoring of *process* in the world really get at the basic question which must, ultimately, relate to level of function, or health status, of the client community. There can be no satisfactory conceptualization of what degree of thoroughness of clinical examination, what utilization of laboratory facilities, what proportion of referrals, what carefulness in record keeping, etc. etc., (all of which are standard parts of process review) is adequate or satisfactory without examining their impact upon the health status of the client population.

UTILIZATION AND DISTRIBUTION

Although there have been many utilization studies, few have been able to incorporate what, according to conventional thinking, ought to be the prime determining factor: health status. Though there have been few distributional studies of health care, those that do exist show how health care (or public health care spending) is distributed according to persons' or families' incomes, not according to health status or need for health care.

Whether or not one takes the rather determined view that the objective of the health services is to make the maximum impact on need, as argued in chapter four, both these limitations are serious. If one *does* accept the view that the health services should make the maximum possible impact on health needs then the limitations are very serious indeed: utilization studies without a health status measure are, at best, merely behavioural studies that omit what, *prima facie*, must be a principal determinant. The omission also means they are quite useless for policy purposes because no inference will be possible concerning whether the 'right' people are getting the care. Distributional studies which are not related to health status will be quite irrelevant since, on this view, the purpose of the health system is not to distribute health care resources to the poor from the rich (absolutely or relatively) but to those, whether rich or poor, who need them.

One recent utilization study in the United States that did incorporate health status variables in the analysis was that of Davis and Reynolds (1975). They found that the number of chronic conditions occurring more than three months prior to the interview, limitations of activity by chronic conditions, and the number of restricted activity days during the preceding two weeks, had a strong positive and highly significant (statistically) impact on the number of physician visits made by those receiving ambulatory care.

The most recent study for Canada is one by Manga for Ontario (Manga, 1976, chap. 6). Unfortunately, this study did not utilize any health status measures as determinants of utilization. He found that physician visits increased with (OHIP) family income, except that the lowest income group (under $5,000 in 1974-5) had more visits than the next highest – a pattern similar to that found by Davis and Reynolds – even after allowing for the effects of family size and other variables (except health status). Davis and Reynolds found that this 'J curve' relating utilization and income disappeared after standardizing for health status and showed a uniform increase instead. Manga believed that one of his variables (a dummy variable taking the value 1 if the family head were retired or disabled and 0 otherwise) appeared to be a proxy for health status – the effect of its addition was to reduce the benefits attributable to low income alone, and hence to 'straighten out' the 'J curve,' and also to reduce the effect attributable to age alone.

Thus, both these studies, Davis and Reynolds directly and Manga indirectly, point to health status (or need) as a significant factor affecting utilization rates. This, of course, is as it should be. The interesting outstanding questions relate to whether, if a more comprehensive definition of health status in terms of functioning were devised, it would explain even a larger part of the variance in utilization that is suggested by these studies, and to what interpretation would remain to be placed upon any residual relationship between income and utilization, or income and public spending on the health care received. It would seem, for example, highly misleading to describe such spending as 'regressive' were it to be found that *utilization* was not dependent significantly upon income, but upon health status, but nevertheless spending was related to income, for even in a perfectly efficient system on the supply side which met only the more urgent needs, if it turned out that the relatively rich had relatively costly illnesses to cure or care for, the apparent 'regressivity' of public spending would be entirely spurious.

Another recent study for Ontario demonstrates dramatically the value of a health status measure in utilization studies. Wolfson and Solari (1976) attempted to identify 'abuse' of physicians' services. Of the various determinants they used to explain utilization the most powerful turned out consistently to be health status, as measured by the Wolfson index. Variables hypothesized to be related to patient-generated abuse (e.g., age and sex) or to doctor-generated abuse (e.g., higher than average cost per patient, given the area and the specialty) had either low explanatory power or low statistical significance. Wolfson and Solari were able to conclude that 'the major determinant of utilization of medical services is ill-health.' Not, perhaps a surprising conclusion, but one to be borne in mind by those advocating deterrent charges on the grounds that patients otherwise demand 'too much' service (Special Program Review, 1975). If there is 'too much' service, the explanation must lie on the 'production' side, for it has no support from the demand side.

From our point of view, the chief value of these illustrative examples is that they show the power of a health status measure in helping to resolve important – and often controversial – issues by shedding factual light on their quantitative significance. If we can agree that the main job of the health services is to prevent and to rectify ill-health, then it is at the least encouraging to find that the evidence, patchy though it is, indicates the right kind of relationship between utilization and need in Ontario. But if we are really to take this objective seriously we have also to ask quite fundamental questions about traditional studies of utilization and distribution. In particular, instead of focusing as intently as has usually been the case upon income in examining regressivity, should not the focus be placed principally upon the association between resources used up and health needs? If that is the proper direction for future distributional studies to take, it does not follow that the association between income (or wealth) and resources use ceases to be of normative interest, but it would reduce it to a status more in keeping with what we believe its true policy significance ought to be.

COST-EFFECTIVENESS OF PROGRAMS

Although there is now no shortage of cost-benefit studies in the health field (see Culyer, Wiseman and Walker, 1977) relatively few explicitly cost or value units of improvement in health status. Most are content with assuming that the outputs of the alternative programs to be evaluated are the same per person (e.g., Piachaud and Weddell, 1972), which begs the question, or with treating the output as life-years gained (e.g., Klarman *et al.*, 1968), which is highly restrictive, since most health care activities are not concerned with the preservation of life, or, in preventive studies, with assessing outcome or treatment costs avoided (e.g., Pole 1971), which again begs an important part of the question. In short, the general tendency is to avoid the difficult but crucial issues involved in measuring, costing, and valuing changes in the health status of patients. The purpose of this section is not to draw particular attention to all the crude calculations made in the name of cost-benefit analysis of health services,[7] but rather to indicate the kind of progress that can be made by using health status measures in cost-benefit type studies. We draw on Torrance's work, outlined in chapter five, as he has applied it to renal failure programs in Ontario.

It has been well-known since Klarman *et al.* (1968) that a ranking of the costliness of kidney transplantation against home and hospital dialysis varies according as one considers the total expenditure per person or per life-year gained. It was recognized in that study, however, that a life-year after transplantation and without dialysis was not quite the 'same' as a life year with dialysis. In fact, Klarman *et al.* considered that a life-year without dialysis was equivalent (in terms of quality of life) to 1.25 years of life with dialysis: a factor precisely the same as that used by the Committee on Chronic Disease in 1967.

The population means, using both the time trade-off and the standard gamble results for his sample, were found by Torrance (1970) to be healthy = 1, kidney transplant = 0.83, home dialysis = 0.66, hospital dialysis = 0.53, dead = 0. It is notable that the ratio of the transplant weight to the home dialysis weight is 1.26. These, when multiplied by the period of time expected to be spent in each state, can then be used to derive outputs for the three programs: outputs for which unit costs may then be calculated.

At first blush, there may appear to be some difficulty in making commensurate the interval scale of these scores with the ratio scale of the monetary measures of the savings from additional earnings by the patients (traditionally counted as a 'benefit' in such studies). Regardless of the validity of this measure of benefit (a validity we doubt) it is useful to recall that the symmetry of benefits foregone (= cost) or costs avoided (= benefit) enables the monetary variables to be grouped together as net costs, leaving that output unvalued in dollars (the life-years weighted by the index scores) as the denominator for the calculation of (net) cost-effectiveness ratios. Using epidemiological data, deriving standardized outputs for each program, and discounting both costs and benefits at 8 per cent, Torrance calculated cost-effectiveness ratios of 177.3 (home dialysis), 16.6 (hospital dialysis), and 255.5 (transplant) per patient.

Although criticism can be levelled at the use of discounted earnings as a benefit and at the inclusion, uncritically, of the direct expenditures on the programs as a valid measure of social cost, Torrance's work demonstrates the

7 For two very different, but equally critical, views and suggestions for the reform of practice as regards the valuation of life-years see Akehurst and Culyer (1975) and Jones-Lee (1976).

feasibility and usefulness of health indexes in cost-benefit type calculations. In grossing-up his per-patient data to program scale, he also exercised more ingenuity than Klarman *et al.* in their (admittedly pioneering) work. Thus, he allowed (roughly) for the probability that the medical-effectiveness of the respective treatments would be worse at the margin than on the average (assuming that patients with the best prognosis are taken first).

Although Torrance (1970, 193) claims that (generalized) cost-effectiveness analysis 'takes over at the point where cost-benefit leaves off,' it will be clear that the technique does *not* enable us to tell whether any transplantation at all should take place, rather that some other (possibly non-health) use of these resources unless it is so general as to become a cost-benefit analysis. Moreover, cost-benefit analysis, even of the 'productive resources' variety criticized by Torrance, can never, given its characteristic methodological foundations, judge any program as 'unacceptable' as Torrance believed, if only by virtue of the fact that benefits are never fully quantified. It can merely identify those, *prima facie*, that *do* pass the efficiency test and those that *may not*. Cost-effectiveness, again given its characteristic methodological foundations, cannot even go this far.

These considerations, however, should not blind us to the fact that Torrance's methodology (which he also applied to other health programs in Ontario) has taken us a good deal further than was previously possible. He has pointed a way towards what ought to become standard practice in the evaluation of health programs in Ontario: if we are not yet at the stage at which it is possible to identify those programs that ought to be adopted, and their appropriate scale, at least we have sufficient knowledge to identify the *prima facie* best programs among a subset, once it has been decided that the output they will produce is to be had.

CONCLUSIONS

Enough will have been said in the foregoing to illustrate the wide applicability of the health index concept in health service planning and monitoring in Ontario. There is, of course, much that has been omitted. For example, we have not discussed the use of the indexes as measures of physician productivity and hence their role in manpower planning. Nor have we discussed their relationship to other measures such as indexes of accessibility (which were proposed in Ontario Council of Health, 1976 and are discussed at length in Aday and Anderson, 1975). Nor have we here explored the many difficult questions associated with the clinical effectiveness of treatments in terms of their tested impact on the natural history of disease.

Our fundamental perspective has remained throughout that health status indexes are *output* measures or *potential output* (need) indexes. The acid test of any health system must remain the extent to which it improves health status over and above what it would otherwise have been. Conventional morbidity and mortality statistics in Ontario are *not* satisfactory substitutes for the real thing: they are arbitrarily weighted, they are often based on process rather than the population at risk, they are hard to relate to specific institutions and health service organizations and they often describe conditions that are unavoidable, persistent, or incurable, at least in the short term.

The ideal must remain to measure *functioning* of individuals: how well a person operates, in his social situation, independently, and without anxiety and pain. The test of the system's effectiveness is whether and how much such functioning is improved. Some of the indexes we have illustrated go only some way towards meeting this specification. For example, Wolfson's pioneering work remains locked into a disease classification base, despite the fact that much medical activity is devoted to the alleviation of side-effects and symptoms, enabling patients to live with their conditions.

Whether we discuss regional allocation, clinical effectiveness, manpower planning, medical research, optimal length of hospital inpatient stay, the objective remains that of a cost-effective health service where both the costs and effects are conceived of in their broadest, humanitarian senses, and not in the philistine cash-accounting terms that the phrase may suggest to some.

It may be asked: 'is there some principle that overrides the basic one that the physician should decide the best service for his patients, should provide it, and is entitled to those resources which would enable him to do so, and be accountable only to his own professional conscience and the views of his professional peers?' The answer is that there is such a principle. It is a principle based on the facts that the resources used for one patient cannot be used for another, and so no individual practitioner can act as though he (with *his* patients) were an island; that some are sick that do not receive care from any physicians; that the public interest in good health, which leads to the government being its principal source of finance, requires not only that its health objectives are accounted for but that health priorities have continuously to be weighed against many other claims on resources. The principle is that, out of a given total budget, we want to make the maximum possible reduction in ill health. While the individual physician must be left free to exercise his best judgment as to the management of his own cases, the resources he uses up in so doing are not free and, in providing them, society has every right to expect that they are used to the best effect. The better society can measure these effects, the less arbitrary the controls it imposes are likely to be.

In this chapter, we have shown some of the tentative steps that have been, and could be, made along this attractive road in Ontario. Although it will be a good many years before systematic measurement of the sort we have discussed becomes routine, and many administrative, political and technical problems remain, the full flowering both of scientific medicine and of rational health service planning and management require it. The indications are, as we have shown, that what is desirable is also practicable. The next steps for Ontario are the subject matter of the last chapter.

7
Regional health patterns in Ontario

The object in this chapter is to examine the data that are currently readily available to see whether it is possible to make any broad generalization about the matching of resources to needs in the province. As we shall see, some associations in the data appear to be consistent with other, more detailed, studies and enable a few broad generalizations. For the most part, however, we shall find that the current information base is grossly inadequate: in general there is no way of telling whether Ontario is successful in attaining its health service objectives whether couched in terms of the language of efficiency, effectiveness, or equity. Consequently, it is not possible to tell whether, in general, health provision in the province is maldistributed.

There are several geographical units that could be used for the comparisons to be made. Few of them are practical for our purposes. Ideally, we could make our examination according to district health units. Apart from the fact that few district health councils have as yet been established, some of our data were not available in ready form for these areas. For example, given the dearth of need indexes, we were anxious to use the Wolfson measures, which would have required recalculation from a county basis to a district basis.

Another possibility would be to examine communities according to their population size, after Dowie *et al.* (Committee on the Healing Arts, 1970, 153-6); however availability of data on this basis again presents difficulties.

The choice has been to gather data by county, regional municipality, territorial district, and census division basis, primarily because vital statistics on births, deaths and so on, are also available on this basis and the Wolfson indexes discussed above are also available for counties. There are problems involved in this choice. For example there are five counties and districts in Ontario which share a municipality with a neighbouring county or district. Health need and provision data collected from such areas are open to distribution by migration over county lines, however this is true of all countries to some extent.

Where possible, more aggregated information about the primary indicators is presented in regional subtotals. The regions chosen are Ministry of Health administrative regions: Northwest, Northeast, Southwest, Central West, Central East, East, and Metro Toronto.

It is important to note, however, that the major conclusions of this chapter are unlikely to be affected by the choice of geographic unit, since the nature of these conclusions is not in the form of an authoritative assessment of current geographical distributions of resources, but to point up why existing data, whatever the basic unit, are inadequate for the task.

The principal criterion for the selection of indexes is that they should be readily available. This enables us to paint a picture of current territorial allocations that identifies major gaps in such data, if reasonable inferences about, for example, the matching of supply to need or the substitution of one kind of resource for another, are to be made.

This drastically reduces the indicators of outcome or need. In principle, what is wanted is a measure of either (a) the potential avoidability of ill-health (prevention potential), or (b) the potential reducibility of ill-health (cure or alleviation potential). None of the four indicators used possesses these characteristics, instead they represent measures of absolute, or relative, ill-health. Moreover, the four indexes used (the two Wolfson indexes, crude mortality and infant mortality) in both original form and related to the provincial average, do not include indexes discussed above and frequently proposed, such as life expectancy at birth, average age at death, prime-age mortality and maternal mortality. These data, while obtainable from the census, are unfortunately not currently available on a county basis. As will be recalled from chapter two, life expectancy at birth and prime-age mortality were proposed by the Economic Council of Canada, while life expectancy at several ages, disability rates, and maternal mortality rates were recommended as indicators by the OECD.

These, then, are the indexes of 'need.' Note that the Wolfson-based measures are subject to the two limitations of process-based measures identified in chapter six: they are based on persons treated rather than persons sick, and they are located by place and treatment rather than residence. It is difficult to know as yet how distorting these factors are. Suffice it to say that the results of the comparisons in this chapter are to be seen as exemplary and illustrative, not as descriptively accurate and prescriptive.

In addition to the four indicators of 'need,' we present indicators of resource availability, divided into three subsets: manpower, hospitals and total expenditures. To facilitate county comparisons, these data were converted to rates per

1000 population or, in the case of expenditures, spending per capita. In this way one obtains a number of rough estimates of availability of resources to individuals in one county, relative to that in another county. This procedure does not, of course, make any allowance for population density. The District of Thunder Bay, for example, has the same number of physicians per 1000 population as Essex County. Clearly, however, the higher concentration of Essex County's inhabitants in a smaller area, makes physicians in that area more readily accessible than in Thunder Bay. This should be kept in mind when interpreting our observations.

The statistics upon which the analysis of the present chapter is based, are presented in their entirety in Tables 18 and 19.

NEED

We have already noted the degree of correlation (or lack of it) between the indexes of ill-health in chapter six. The correlations between the complete set presented in this chapter are shown in Table 20.

Here it can be seen that, as one would expect, there is a strong, statistically significant correlation between the two sets of Wolfson indexes. While the hospital health indexes are not significantly correlated with either crude or perinatal mortality rates, the claims index has a fairly strong correlation with crude mortality rates (significant at the 99.9 per cent level of confidence). Not surprisingly, crude mortality rates are significantly correlated with perinatal mortality rates. The absence of correlation between the hospital indexes and mortality may be due to migration of patients across boundaries: whether this is so must, however, be largely a matter for speculation at present.

The regional distribution of morbidity and mortality, according to our four sets of indicators, has been shown in Table 18. We have not weighted and combined them to form a single over-all indicator. There are at least four reasons for this. Firstly, the construction of any weighted index would involve us in making arbitrary (from a policy view) value judgments. Secondly, the indexes do not measure entirely different elements of ill-health, for example, crude mortality includes perinatal mortality; mortality is included in the Wolfson indexes; patients treated both in hospital and by a primary physician count twice in the Wolfson indexes. Thirdly, some indexes are inherently correlated with provision indicators. For example, Wolfson's indexes are based upon hospital throughput or primary physician's throughput and it is not surprising to find them correlated with the supply of physicians, dentists, RNs, staffed beds, hospital services expenditures, and physicians services expenditures. Finally, the

TABLE 18

Indicators of need for health services

County	(1)	(1a)	(2)	(2a)	(3)	(3a)	(4)	(4a)
Essex	3.57	−0.20	75	0.34	8.13	0.08	22.1	0.13
Kent	4.65	0.04	70	0.25	8.91	0.18	22.0	0.13
Lambton	3.93	−0.12	68	0.21	8.04	0.07	22.9	0.17
Bruce	3.40	−0.24	66	0.18	10.21	0.35	14.7	−0.25
Grey	5.52	0.24	82	0.46	10.46	0.39	21.7	0.11
Huron	5.07	0.14	76	0.36	10.85	0.44	16.8	−0.14
Perth	4.34	−0.03	59	0.05	9.51	0.26	23.7	0.22
Middlesex	7.10	0.59	79	0.41	7.33	−0.03	16.7	−0.14
Oxford	5.77	0.29	76	0.36	9.03	0.20	19.2	−0.02
Elgin	4.48	0.00	69	0.23	9.52	0.26	19.4	−0.01
SOUTH WESTERN REGION	4.97	0.11	74	0.32	8.46	0.12	20.0	0.03
Wellington	4.24	−0.05	61	0.09	7.61	0.01	19.7	0.01
Dufferin	5.01	0.12	38	−0.32	9.01	0.19	31.8	0.03
Waterloo	2.79	−0.37	59	0.05	6.29	−0.17	19.3	−0.01
Halton	3.78	−0.15	48	−0.14	4.92	−0.35	6.8	−0.14
Brant	5.83	0.31	84	0.50	8.77	0.16	20.6	0.86
Hamilton/ Wentworth	6.17	0.38	78	0.39	7.75	0.03	17.8	−0.09
Haldimand/ Norfolk	3.56	−0.20	72	0.29	10.15	0.29	24.1	0.24
Niagara	4.89	0.10	72	0.29	7.99	0.06	21.2	0.09
CENTRAL WEST REGION	4.63	0.04	67	0.20	7.20	−0.05	18.3	−0.06

Muskoka	3.23	−0.28	52	−0.07	10.57	0.40	24.0	0.23
Haliburton	3.98	−0.11	47	−0.16	11.17	0.48	29.9	0.53
Simcoe	4.34	−0.03	40	−0.29	8.92	0.18	18.6	−0.05
Victoria	6.59	0.48	77	0.38	11.39	0.51	16.3	−0.16
Peterborough	6.19	0.39	76	0.36	8.94	0.19	24.6	0.26
Peel	2.26	−0.49	28	−0.50	3.94	−0.48	15.7	−0.19
Durham	3.22	−0.28	44	−0.21	6.96	−0.08	19.4	0.00
Northumberland	1.60	−0.64	60	0.07	9.45	0.25	22.6	0.13
York	5.03	0.13	40	−0.29	7.59	0.01	18.7	−0.04
Metro Toronto	5.22	0.17	40	−0.29	7.08	−0.06	18.3	−0.06
CENTRAL EAST REGION	4.68	0.05	41	−0.27	6.92	−0.08	18.4	−0.06
Hastings	5.15	0.15	83	0.48	9.03	0.20	17.8	−0.09
Prince Edward	1.42	−0.68	77	0.38	11.84	0.57	25.3	0.30
Renfrew	3.86	−0.13	55	−0.02	7.92	0.05	21.9	0.12
Lennox & Addington	2.12	−0.52	45	−0.20	7.88	0.05	21.4	0.10
Frontenac	6.79	0.52	89	0.59	7.30	−0.03	18.7	−0.06
Lanark	5.71	0.28	88	0.57	11.45	0.52	26.1	0.34
Leeds & Grenville	3.46	−0.19	63	0.13	9.79	0.30	23.2	0.21
Ottawa-Carleton	2.76	−0.38	61	0.09	6.85	−0.09	19.6	0.01
Prescott & Russell	2.55	−0.43	66	0.17	8.44	0.12	28.0	0.43
Stormont/Dundas/ Glengarry	5.39	0.21	69	0.23	9.84	0.31	25.3	0.30

TABLE 18, *continued*

Indicators of need for health services

County	(1)	(1a)	(2)	(2a)	(3)	(3a)	(4)	(4a)
EASTERN REGION	3.81	-0.15	67	0.20	7.87	0.04	21.0	0.08
Algoma	3.96	-0.11	53	-0.05	6.42	-0.15	18.3	-0.06
Cochrane	3.66	-0.18	55	-0.02	7.57	0.00	24.7	0.27
Sudbury	2.47	-0.45	48	-0.14	5.47	-0.27	21.6	0.11
Timiskaming	3.88	-0.13	57	0.01	9.82	0.30	26.1	0.34
Manitoulin	2.04	-0.54	54	-0.04	11.80	0.56	17.9	-0.08
Parry Sound	4.50	0.01	81	0.45	10.23	0.37	20.6	0.06
Nipissing	3.86	-0.13	57	0.02	7.68	0.02	23.1	0.18
NORTH EASTERN Region	3.38	-0.24	54	-0.04	6.97	-0.08	21.8	0.12
Kenora	2.84	-0.36	44	-0.21	8.44	0.12	21.0	0.08
Rainy River	5.38	0.21	62	0.11	9.22	0.22	30.0	0.54
Thunder Bay	4.79	0.07	56	0.00	9.85	0.20	16.2	-0.17
NORTH WESTERN REGION	4.34	-0.03	53	-0.05	8.89	0.18	18.5	-0.05
ONTARIO	4.46	–	56	–	7.54	–	19.5	–

NOTES: (1) Wolfson's hospital health index (1972-3); (1a) Wolfson's hospital health index (1972-3) – relative to Ontario provincial average; (2) Wolfson's claims health index (1972-3); (2a) Wolfson's claims health index (1972-3) – relative to Ontario provincial average; (3) Number of deaths per 1000 population (1973); (3a) Number of deaths per 1000 population (1973) – relative to Ontario provincial average; (4) Number of perinatal deaths per 1000 births, including stillbirths (1972-3 average); (4a) Number of perinatal deaths per 1000 births, including stillbirths (1972-3 average) – relative to Ontario provincial average.

TABLE 19

Indicators of health services provision and expenditure

County	(6)	(7)	(8)	(9)	(10)	(11)	(12)	(13)
Essex	1.29	0.33	6.02	1.71	5.99	6.42	134.03	72.94
Kent	1.07	0.32	6.45	2.60	8.47	5.92	112.93	58.27
Lambton	1.27	0.33	6.37	2.59	7.07	5.68	112.10	66.27
Bruce	0.83	0.31	5.42	3.17	10.40	5.69	78.16	36.47
Grey	1.38	0.41	6.78	3.80	7.67	7.33	138.59	68.30
Huron	0.96	0.31	5.43	4.92	10.77	6.27	103.00	37.80
Perth	1.22	0.34	6.45	2.63	7.43	7.02	126.89	52.84
Middlesex	2.79	0.58	8.85	3.71	4.50	7.70	244.36	95.57
Oxford	1.17	0.36	5.61	2.88	7.27	5.29	104.17	51.39
Elgin	1.06	0.25	6.40	5.96	11.64	5.28	93.34	46.49
SOUTH WESTERN REGION	1.58	0.39	6.79	3.05	6.22	6.52	145.51	69.21
Wellington	1.27	0.35	6.47	2.54	7.07	5.22	107.83	65.91
Dufferin	0.86	0.34	4.94	2.58	8.74	5.92	88.26	42.85
Waterloo	1.23	0.43	5.28	1.55	5.58	5.28	110.81	62.48
Halton	1.57	0.80	6.41	1.69	5.15	4.42	88.74	66.23
Brant	1.14	0.29	6.01	2.83	7.73	6.49	132.44	68.33
Hamilton-Wentworth	2.01	0.46	6.06	2.83	4.43	6.74	208.57	85.70
Haldimand-Norfolk	0.77	0.28	4.63	2.53	9.35	4.60	76.67	49.73
Niagara	1.26	0.38	5.31	1.94	5.76	5.76	109.40	68.24
CENTRAL WEST REGION	1.45	0.45	5.73	2.21	5.49	5.69	131.47	69.83
Muskoka	1.27	0.46	5.53	2.65	6.45	5.01	97.48	48.49
Haliburton	0.85	0.21	2.87	1.28	4.88	2.13	28.49	26.05
Simcoe	1.27	0.37	5.60	2.68	6.54	4.61	84.04	56.00
Victoria	1.23	0.30	5.11	2.02	5.78	3.23	90.59	51.91

TABLE 19, *continued*

Indicators of health services provision and expenditure

County	(6)	(7)	(8)	(9)	(10)	(11)	(12)	(13)
Peterborough	1.58	0.49	7.20	2.57	6.17	6.06	142.85	81.15
Peel	1.28	0.18	5.52	1.51	5.48	2.88	60.54	69.36
Durham	1.24	0.35	1.22	2.75	3.19	4.47	98.27	67.52
Northumberland	0.68	0.19	3.79	1.81	8.24	5.05	89.91	29.47
York	1.38	0.58	6.05	1.48	5.46	2.43	171.76	94.49
Metro Toronto	2.35	0.58	6.33	1.40	5.40	6.84	*	*
CENTRAL EAST REGION	1.97	0.50	5.78	1.65	3.78	5.77	146.15	85.12
Hastings	1.31	0.35	5.84	1.52	5.64	6.63	126.58	63.18
Prince Edward	0.98	0.23	4.81	3.13	8.10	4.44	55.11	27.69
Renfrew	0.88	0.34	6.11	2.20	9.51	6.15	108.66	40.34
Lennox & Addington	0.84	0.10	5.02	2.35	8.81	2.51	41.43	24.21
Frontenac	3.76	0.40	9.56	3.51	3.47	9.81	291.14	100.05
Lanark	1.32	0.38	8.07	5.72	10.46	8.05	150.48	50.41
Leeds & Grenville	1.47	0.36	8.05	5.00	8.93	4.25	88.84	48.18
Ottawa-Carleton	2.41	0.53	7.15	1.34	3.52	6.38	149.79	78.98
Prescott & Russell	0.93	0.13	2.41	1.48	4.18	1.61	27.29	28.56
Stormont/Dundas/ Glengary	1.11	0.20	6.61	2.01	– 7.72	7.03	138.65	49.94
EASTERN REGION	1.96	0.40	6.92	2.18	4.64	6.35	143.00	66.10
Algoma	1.16	0.28	5.41	2.17	6.56	6.36	124.97	43.36
Cochrane	0.87	0.20	4.48	2.13	7.56	5.68	104.35	48.81
Sudbury	0.95	0.25	4.27	2.07	6.53	5.34	101.13	54.31
Timiskaming	1.08	0.20	5.56	3.24	8.15	8.63	127.43	46.49
Manitoulin	0.57	0.09	4.25	2.55	12.00	7.64	131.26	28.81

	(6)	(7)	(8)	(9)	(10)	(11)	(12)	(13)
Parry Sound	1.35	0.22	4.94	4.29	6.86	6.96	139.53	46.60
Nipissing	1.15	0.32	5.64	4.03	8.41	6.34	128.82	51.75
NORTH EASTERN REGION	1.03	0.25	4.86	2.58	7.21	5.78	114.89	49.33
Kenora	0.85	0.24	4.71	3.38	9.52	6.17	109.8	37.24
Rainy River	1.49	0.25	5.08	5.58	7.17	7.19	116.33	43.38
Thunder Bay	1.28	0.40	6.69	4.41	8.70	8.24	164.51	66.82
NORTH WESTERN REGION	1.20	0.34	6.04	4.29	8.63	7.63	146.03	57.11
Ontario	1.72	0.44	6.02	2.19	4.78	6.00	140.43	73.67

NOTES: * included in York County; (6) Number of active physicians per 1000 population (1974); (7) number of active licensed dentists per 1000 population (1974); (8) number of registered nurses employed in nursing, per 1000 population (1974); (9) number of registered nursing assistants employed in nursing, per 1000 population (1974); (10) ratio of RNs and RNAs to physicians (1974); (11) number of staffed public general and allied special hospital beds per 1000 population (1974); (12) Expenditures per capita on hospital services by Ontario Ministry of Health (1974); (13) OHIP payments per capita for claims for physician services (fiscal year 1973-4).

TABLE 20

Correlations of health need indicators

Indicator	(1)	(1a)	(2)	(2a)	(3)	(3a)	(4)	(4a)
(1) Wolfson's hospital health index (1972-3)	1.0000							
(1a) Wolfson's hospital health index rel. to prov. ave.	0.9998 (s = 0.001)	1.0000						
(2) Wolfson's claims health index (1972-3)	0.5029 (s = 0.001)	0.5038 (s = 0.001)	1.0000					
(2a) Wolfson's claims health index rel. to prov. ave.	0.5026 (s = 0.001)	0.5035 (s = 0.001)	0.9999 (s = 0.001)	1.0000				
(3) Crude mortality rate per 1000 pop. (1973)	0.1137 (s = 0.221)	0.1146 (s = 0.219)	0.4283 (s = 0.001)	0.4280 (s = 0.001)	1.0000			
(3a) Crude mortality rate rel. to prov. ave.	0.1191 (s = 0.210)	0.1201 (s = 0.208)	0.4311 (s = 0.001)	0.4307 (s = 0.001)	0.9993 (s = 0.001)	1.0000		
(4) Perinatal mortality rate per 1000 births (1972-3)	-0.0794 (s = 0.296)	-0.0790 (s =0.297)	0.0204 (s = 0.445)	0.0190 (s = 0.449)	0.3906 (s = 0.003)	0.3888 (s = 0.003)	1.0000	
(4a) Perinatal mortality rate rel. to prov. ave.	-0.0973 (s = 0.255)	-0.0947 (s = 0.261)	-0.1824 (s = 0.107)	-0.1811 (s = 0.109)	0.0202 (s = 0.446)	0.0175 (s = 0.453)	0.2479 (s = 0.045)	1.0000

procedure of combining into one index masks the fact that need may be specific. For example, high perinatal mortality implies a need for better obstetrical and maternity services, not more psychiatric services. For all these measures, it has seemed best to identify the need indexes individually.

Wolfson's hospital index (see Tables 18 and 19) shows a particularly high correlation with health services provision, especially the supply of staffed beds. Areas with a high number of beds per 1000 population also tend to have high rates of ill-health. The same holds with regard to the relationship between Wolfson's indexes, and other provision indicators. In general, Wolfson's indexes show Northern Ontario, notably the districts of Kenora, Cochrane, Algoma, Sudbury, and Manitoulin, to be more healthy than many areas of Southern Ontario (with the possible exception of the Central East Region, and Renfrew and Lennox-Addington counties). One must be wary of inferring that this is a true reflection of the general levels of health in these counties, however, since they are also among those with low provision levels. Nor should one infer that increases in provision in these areas of apparently good health are unjustified. The association between regional health status, as measured by the Wolfson index, and provision levels is to be expected, not from any prior theory of disease prevalence but simply because *the Wolfson indexes are based upon patients processed*, not the population at risk, and to individual *events* in care rather than individual *persons*. Once again we have a result which may be largely attributable to the process-basis of the Wolfson indexes.

If one were to assume that the effect on case-load of increasing hospital beds is not entirely offset by falling occupancy or increasing length of stay, or that increasing physician numbers does not generate a proportionate reduction in case-load per physician – highly realistic assumptions – then it follows with compelling arithmetic force that changes in provision will affect 'need' on the Wolfson index in the same direction. Process-based indexes are quite inappropriate for evaluating the adequacy of geographical resource distribution.

The point is brought out well by a comparison of the correlation between the Wolfson indexes and provision, and the mortality indexes and provision. Table 23 demonstrates that (with the exception of RNA-associated provision indicators, of which more below) the mortality data are *inversely* related to provision levels: in general, areas of high 'need' are also areas of low provision. It is not necessary, of course, to remind the reader of the gross inadequacy of mortality as a measure of the need for health services. Nor should one forget that health services are but one of a set of factors affecting health status on the one hand and but one, therefore, of a set of factors which may be used to affect changes in health status. Neither causal affect nor policy implication should therefore be read into these associations.

The crude death rate for Ontario was 7.54 in 1973 per 1,000 and its distribution is given in Table 18. Not surprisingly, the urban areas of Southern Ontario appear to fare better than other parts of the province. London-Middlesex, Halton, Peel, Waterloo, Metro Toronto, Kingston-Frontenac, and Ottawa-Carleton have rates below the provincial average, along with Sudbury and Algoma.

The fourth indicator is perinatal mortality. This is defined as stillbirths (over 28 weeks) plus infant deaths (under 7 days old), divided by the total number of births (including stillbirths). This is usually regarded as a good measure of pre-natal and early post-natal health and quality of care.

Distribution of perinatal mortality within Ontario is illustrated in Table 18, which also shows that eighteen counties had rates below the provincial mean (when averaged over the two-year 1972-3 period). Of this number, only two, Thunder Bay and Manitoulin, are found in the north.

PROVISION

The criteria we would ideally wish to use imply that area resource allocation should relate to those area health needs that are capable of amelioration by health service provision. There are many difficulties at present in making this relationship. Some, as we have seen above, relate to our available measures of need. Others come mainly from the supply side.

One of the first is that residents of one region who require health care may cross into another to obtain it. Similarly, health care personnel, resident in one locality, may in fact be employed in another. In either event the available statistics may distort the normal relationship between local supply and need. More fundamental are the problems of interpreting the apparent relationships between supply and need. For example, it is obviously not always the case that the provision of more hospital beds is the appropriate response to more illness in a given area. More appropriate supply responses might rather be to increase preventive health services, or reduce length of stay, or increase primary care services. There is also uncertainty about how some inputs can be substituted for others. For instance, as will be pointed out below, there is evidence to suggest that there is substitution of registered nurses and nursing assistants for physicians in poorer, rural and remote areas. Whether the higher death rates in these areas are attributable to such substitution or the substitution is a response to rates that would otherwise be higher still, cannot be established from these data alone.

Another consideration that must be reckoned with is that there may be economies or diseconomies of scale in the provision of some health services. In the case of the former, highly populous communities may be expected to require a lower per capita endowment to achieve the same impact on community health status while, in the case of the latter, the converse would be expected.

Finally, there is a kind of 'regression fallacy.' If we conceive health resources as meeting (and hence reducing) need, then the temptation to deplore a negative association between needs and resources (even if they were measured more satisfactorily than is at present possible) should be resisted. The problem arises essentially because of the static nature of the data used. Ideally, the criterion should relate to the *change* in health status associated with *changes* in resource provision, not to extant levels of status and provision. Absolute levels of need in the community, and absolute levels of provision are extremely crude indicators of where resources ought to go. High needs that are not amenable to treatment or prevention, or that are relatively costly to treat or prevent, are not necessarily high priorities. High levels of resource provision, whose productivity at the margin is relatively high, are not necessarily low priorities for extension.

Many of these problems can be illustrated using the available data. Table 21 correlates the entire set of provision indicators, and these are then correlated with the principal need indicators in Tables 22 and 23.

Table 21 shows that nearly all primary provision indicators are significantly correlated with each other. In particular, the supply of dentists is strongly correlated with the supply of physicians and RNs, as well as with expenditures on hospital and physician services. As one might expect, the supplies of physicians and RNs are correlated with each other as well as with the supply of staffed beds and expenditures on hospital and physician services.

Dentists, physicians, and RNs tend to be concentrated in areas where hospitals and other medical facilities are present. Most notably, in Northern Ontario (with the exception of Timiskaming, Parry Sound, and Manitoulin) where there is a relative scarcity of dentists, physicians and RNs, we also observe a low rate of hospital bed provision. There is also some evidence of substitution of RNs and especially RNAs for physicians in these same areas. We might note in particular, the strong negative correlations between the ratio of RNs and RNAs to physicians, and the supplies of physicians and dentists, as well as expenditures on hospital and physician services.

The regional distribution of the two major components of the health service dollar can be deduced from Table 19. Comparison with distribution of crude mortality rate and perinatal death rate (see Table 18) shows that areas like Middlesex, Wentworth, York, Metro Toronto, Frontenac, Lanark, and Thunder Bay, which have high per capita expenditures on hospital and physicians services, also generally have lower mortality rates (with the exceptions of Lanark and Thunder Bay). Meanwhile, areas like Haliburton, Victoria, and the counties

TABLE 21

Correlations of health provision and expenditure indicators

Indicator	(6)	(7)	(8)	(9)	(10)	(11)	(12)	(13)
(6) Active physicians per 1000 population (1974)	1.0000							
(7) Active licensed dentists per 1000 population (1974)	0.5812 (s = 0.001)	1.0000						
(8) RNs employed in nursing per 1000 population (1974)	0.6532 (s = 0.001)	0.5039 (s = 0.001)	1.0000					
(9) RNAs employed in nursing per 1000 population (1974)	0.0656 (s = 0.329)	−0.0869 (s = 0.278)	0.3245 (s = 0.012)	1.0000				
(10) Ratio of RNs & RNAs to physicians (1974)	−0.5872 (s = 0.001)	−0.4221 (s = 0.001)	0.0286 (s = 0.424)	0.5225 (s = 0.001)	1.0000			
(11) Staffed beds per 1000 population (1974)	0.4163 (s = 0.002)	0.1463 (s = 0.161)	0.5357 (s = 0.001)	0.4203 (s = 0.001)	0.1785 (s = 0.112)	1.0000		
(12) Expenditures per capita on hospital services (1974)	0.7810 (s = 0.001)	0.4485 (s = 0.001)	0.6724 (s = 0.001)	0.2318 (s = 0.058)	−0.2434 (s = 0.050)	0.7340 (s = 0.001)	1.0000	
(13) Expenditures per capita on physician services (1973-4)	0.7604 (s = 0.001)	0.6918 (s = 0.001)	0.5720 (s = 0.001)	−0.0912 (s = 0.271)	−0.5782 (s = 0.001)	0.2937 (s = 0.023)	0.7418 (s = 0.001)	1.0000

TABLE 22

Correlations of health provision and expenditure indicators with health need indicators

Indicator	Wolfson's hosp. health index (1972-3)	Wolfson's claims health index (1972-3)	Crude mortality rate (1973)	Perinatal mortality rate (1972-3)	Days of care given per capita (1974)
Active physicians per 1000 population (1974)	0.5245 ($s = 0.001$)	0.2762 ($s = 0.029$)	0.3302 ($s = 0.011$)	0.2719 ($s = 0.031$)	0.5272 ($s = 0.001$)
Active licensed dentists per 1000 population (1974)	0.4263 ($s = 0.001$)	0.0307 ($s = 0.418$)	-0.3438 ($s = 0.008$)	-0.4582 ($s = 0.001$)	0.2229 ($s = 0.064$)
RNs employed in nursing per 1000 population (1974)	0.5503 ($s = 0.001$)	0.4075 ($s = 0.002$)	-0.0683 ($s = 0.322$)	-0.2371 ($s = 0.052$)	0.6155 ($s = 0.001$)
RNAs employed in nursing per 1000 population (1974)	0.2856 ($s = 0.025$)	0.3651 ($s = 0.005$)	0.4014 ($s = 0.002$)	0.1106 ($s = 0.227$)	0.3637 ($s = 0.006$)
Ratio of RNs and RNAs to physicians (1974)	-0.1834 ($s = 0.106$)	0.0508 ($s = 0.366$)	0.5251 ($s = 0.001$)	0.1286 ($s = 0.192$)	0.0662 ($s = 0.327$)
Staffed beds per 1000 population (1974)	0.4275 ($s = 0.001$)	0.4254 ($s = 0.001$)	0.1158 ($s = 0.217$)	-0.0342 ($s = 0.409$)	0.9673 ($s = 0.001$)
Expenditures per capita on hospital services (1974)	0.6226 ($s = 0.001$)	0.4348 ($s = 0.001$)	-0.1413 ($s = 0.172$)	-0.2388 ($s = 0.053$)	0.7906 ($s = 0.001$)
Expenditures per capita on physician services (1973/74)	0.5506 ($s = 0.001$)	0.2314 ($s = 0.059$)	-0.4786 ($s = 0.001$)	-0.3756 ($s = 0.005$)	0.4190 ($s = 0.002$)

bordering on Georgian Bay and Lake Huron, have lower-than-average rates of per capita health expenditure, accompanied by higher-than-average mortality rates.

We have already discussed some of the hazards in interpreting the policy significance of the negative correlations between mortality and provision. What conditions would have to be met if we were to infer that the balance of resource distribution ought to be tipped in favour of the high mortality areas? Let us assume that mortality is an adequate descriptor of need. Let us also assume that health service provision is the appropriate way of meeting this need. Moreover, assume that health service provision is the appropriate way of meeting this need (rather than, say, more vigorous anti-poverty measures, housing programs, or public health prevention measures). Let us also assume that the composition of mortality by, say cause of death, gives us an adequate idea of the kind of health service resources that are needed. Then, granted these assumptions, it would still *not* follow that a redistribution of resources away from the low mortality areas towards the high would reduce *over-all* mortality (need, on our assumptions) *unless* the marginal productivity of the transferred resources was higher in the high mortality areas than in the low. Or instead of thinking in terms of redistribution of resources, consider a net increment in resources: the maximum impact of these resources upon over-all mortality would *not* imply that they should go to the areas of highest mortality *unless* their marginal productivity in reducing mortality is highest there.

Even if the proportionate contribution to mortality of each cause of death were the same in high and low mortality areas, it would not follow that the marginal productivity of health service resources was the same in each. The productivity of an additional dollar of spending is affected also by the local prices of resources, by population density, by the lifestyle of the population at risk and by a host of other factors which are at present imperfectly understood in terms of their impact on changing mortality and morbidity, let alone a properly constructed measure of social functioning.

PROVISION AND INCOME LEVELS

It is frequently supposed that family incomes are negatively associated with health status and positively correlated with resource availability. Utilization studies, as we have seen in chapter six, commonly find, even after adjusting for variables such as family size and health status, that utilization and income are positively associated. These effects reveal themselves in the county comparisons made here.

Table 23 shows that mortality indicators, along with the Wolfson claims index, are negatively correlated with income, so areas with higher per capita

TABLE 23

Pearson correlation coefficients of per capita income with 'need' and provision

'Need' and income

Wolfson's hospital health index	WHHL relative to provincial average	Wolfson's claims health index	WCHI relative to provincial average	Crude mortality rate	CMR relative to provincial average	Perinatal mortality rate	PMR relative to provincial average	Days of care given
0.0754 (0.307)	0.0741 (0.310)	−0.2349 (0.056)	−0.2329 (0.058)	−0.8259 (0.001)	−0.8258 (0.001)	−0.4921 (0.001)	−0.0226 (0.440)	0.107 (0.237)

Provision and income

Physicians	Dentists	RNs	RNAs	RNs + RNAs Physicians	Staffed Beds	Expenditure on hospital services	Expenditure on physician services
0.4330 (0.001)	0.5603 (0.001)	0.2307 (0.059)	−0.2638 (0.037)	−0.4972 (0.001)	0.0306 (0.419)	0.3281 (0.012)	0.6957 (0.001)

income, according to the above figures, tend to have less ill health (the Wolfson hospital index is positively associated with income, but then so is hospital provision). The second part of Table 23 bears out the findings of utilization studies – the supply of dentists, physicians, and RNs, along with expenditures on hospital and physician services, are all positively correlated with the level of income per capita. The fact that the ratio of RNs and RNAs to physicians is negatively correlated with income, appears again to be a reflection of the substitution of RNAs for physicians in the poorer, more northerly counties of the province.

Judging from most of the statistics presented in this chapter, it would appear that high income areas are generally in the more densely populated parts of Southern Ontario. Rural and northern areas seem to have fewer facilities and services available to their residents, while outlying and remote regions have problems of accessibility compounded by distance and poor transportation. This distribution problem has been noted in the past (e.g., Mustard Report, 1974; OEC, 1976) and is in large part the consequence of an inheritance from a past in which income was a prime determinant of health resource location. The fascinating question is, of course, how long it will be before a new pattern, now that the market link between income and supply has been thoroughly broken, will emerge or whether the old pattern will maintain itself via the political 'market place.' There can be rather little hope for change unless we face up to the question of measuring both the needs of districts and the productivity of resources in meeting them.

CONCLUSIONS

The examination of this chapter highlights rather clearly the limitations of currently available data for making sensible, if broadly based, decisions about the rationality of area resource distribution in the province. It is plain that measures of ill health based upon process, or throughput, data are not at all suitable for this task: they can give the impression that increased provision increases ill health – a view from which even the more skeptical commentators on the size of the marginal productivity of health services or those that worry most about the increased incidence of iatrogenic disease (Illich apart) would dissent.

But it is also plain that the readily available measures of ill health based on the wider community have severe limitations. First, these mortality data are extremely crude indicators of ill health in developed communities, nor is it appropriate to consider the bulk of day-to-day medical practice to be typically concerned with 'life or death.' Second, static data describing states rather than transitions from one state to another, whether for individuals or for whole populations, can be misleading indicators of priority: if a transition from one state to another can be achieved only at substantially greater cost in one area compared with another, then both humanitarian and financial considerations *may* lead us rationally to prefer to maintain a pattern of regional imbalance in health status. Thirdly, although the Wolfson process-based indexes suffer from the fatal flaw for regional allocation purposes of being process-based, they are nevertheless, in principle, more sensitive measures of the ill health of those whose status they measure. But they still do not measure what we have argued to be the proper basis for ill health measurement, namely the ability of individuals to function normally, and without pain or anxiety, in society.

We conclude that if a rational allocation policy is to be devised for Ontario, then the first essential is for a new data base to be established for the measurement of need. This must be a *community*-based measure of individual functioning capable of being related to the cause(s) of impairment in functioning. It is as simple, but as radically different from current practice, as that!

8

Health status measurement
and health care planning in Ontario

The central theme of this work has been to *identify* the central piece of information that is needed for running an efficient and humane health system in Ontario, given the aspirations outlined in chapter three, and to explore problems of *interpreting* it, *operationalizing* it, and *utilizing* it. This central piece of information concerns, of course, the health status of Ontario residents, and it is a piece of information that we do not currently have.

It would clearly have been well beyond the scope of the present study to have explored, or to have evaluated, past and present health policies and the instruments used to give effect to policies. Chapter seven was not a critique of the ministry's 'underserviced area' program — though it emphasized the lack of suitable performance measures without which such an evaluation is impossible. Chapter six was not a critique of Ontario policy with regard to, say, medical research funding or monitoring clinical practice — rather it attempted to illustrate, using the imperfect data available, how health status measurement can help to inform policy.

In this chapter we continue the emphasis on information rather than actual policy and policy instruments, but since there has to be a *policy about information* we shall inescapably be drawn into making some recommendations. In order to show how these flow from our preceding argument and its illustrations, we first review the principal threads of the argument. We then turn to our recommendations.

THE STORY SO FAR

In the overview of chapter two we looked at some of the general rationales that have been put for health status 'indicators' and 'indexes' with particular attention being given to the cases made by the Economic Council of Canada and the Organization for Economic Cooperation and Development, of which Canada is a member. This served to focus attention from the beginning on these measures as aids to policy-making rather than mere social commenting. We also associated the commonly used expressions health 'indicator' and 'index' broadly with macrocosmic and microcosmic concepts and uses but, while the macro-micro distinction is a useful one, the terms 'indicator' and 'index' were subsequently dropped in favour of a more general term, 'health status measure,' emphasizing the features common to both macro and micro concepts. The OECD proposals for specific measures were described and although their proposals cover more dimensions for evaluating health service efficiency than have been discussed here (including, as they do, measures of 'accessibility' for example), the emphasis on 'ability to function' and on a *community* rather than an *institutional* source for the data was highly applauded and interpreted as consistent with both the Canadian federal government's document *A New Perspective on the Health of Canadians* (Lalonde, 1974) and some of the main ideas behind the proposed Canada Health Survey.

Chapter two also noted that a principal reason for the rising interest from all quarters in health status measurement arises from the steadily increasing involvement of governments in health service provision. Since government and government agencies are among the principal clients for the information provided by health status measurement, chapter three attempts to explain the common intellectual foundation, using the concepts of economics, of both the rationale for governmental intervention in health and for health status measurement.

The basic argument is that the health activities of individuals create what are referred to here as 'spillovers' or what frequently are termed 'externalities' or 'external effects.' Without the jargon this amounts to a recognition by economists that no man is an island. Although there remain those who still maintain that men are sufficiently islands for governments to content themselves (and their subjects) with only the basic peace-keeping activities of a *laissez-faire* state, the arguments against it are really overwhelming – and the evidence of intervention from democratic countries is rather awkward evidence for those who claim that citizens' interest in health are best served by government keeping well away.

The analytical arguments are, however, the ones that chiefly concern us here and in chapter four we identified five 'spillover' effects of importance, the first a basically 'selfish' spillover and the others deriving from what may be termed 'altruistic' sources. The first is the spillover effects of preventing communicable disease; A chooses to become protected (e.g., immunized or improves his own sanitation) and confers a benefit on B in the form of a reduced probability of contracting disease. Since A would normally act only on his own selfish interests and not on B's (equally selfish) interests, he would not count B's benefit in his decision. The consequence is a rate of immunization or public health protection that is generally recognized to be too low; hence government subsidy and/or direct provision.

The other arguments lead analytically in the same direction, though they rest on the observation that people care about one another in various ways. Thus, there are some persons who are recognized to be not very good at taking care of themselves (e.g., young children, some mentally sick, some elderly persons, those too sick to make decisions for themselves) and who 'need,' everyone agrees, community support. It is also clear that people care about the financial burden that ill health can become, even with insurance, but especially for the uninsurable. People care also about the geographical distribution of health care: geographical 'needs' differ and so, the feeling is, should the distribution of resources. Finally, most important for our purposes, and underlying the previous considerations, there is overwhelming evidence that people (or at least those who speak for them) actually care a great deal about the health status of individuals other than themselves.

Our interpretation of these 'spillovers' is that, taken together, they imply that the individuals who make up the community collectively aspire to make receipt of health care independent of ability to pay for it but, indeed, to make it equally available to those in 'need.' Economic analysis thus actually lends its support to those unfortunates who, from their wholly sociological-cum-administrative stances (or, so they are often perceived by economists, who pride themselves on their hard-headedness and intellectual rigour) urged the language of 'need' upon us. It also, as we see in chapter four, provides us with a precise definition. Economics, it turns out, is not stuck with fighting a perpetual rearguard action in defence of the market, and economists ought to be in the vanguard of attempts to banish the final cobwebs from the fuzzy notions of their far-too-frequently-scorned brethren in other social sciences.

Chapter four then brought us to the heart of the matter. The need for health care is there defined in terms of (a) *the potential for avoidance of reductions in health status*, and (b) *the potential for improvements in health status*. With the final emergence of the central character in the plot, the stage is set in chapter four for the analysis of both the concept of health status and the means of altering it. Beginning from a rather stylized notion of 'top-level' choice between 'education' and 'health' the analysis is refined to identify the crucial conceptual problems inescapably involved in defining health status and the effectiveness (or otherwise) of means of affecting it: the potential for change.

This analysis raised questions of value which were systematically addressed in chapter five in the context of a survey of the most interesting attempts that have been made to date to measure health status. Although the argument of this chapter is at times somewhat technical, its chief conclusions are really rather straightforward: controversy about the more sophisticated issues of value need not deter us from making an early start on community health status measurement. There are, to be sure, difficult questions of value involved in compiling a single measure of health status, whether for macro or micro use, and these we shall address in the second part of this concluding chapter.

The next two chapters turned to the application of health status measurement in Ontario, looking at regional comparisons in each — but particularly in chapter seven — and at more micro uses in research priority-setting, quality of care assessment, and cost-effectiveness type studies. Although these examples by no means exhaust the potential illustrations of the usefulness of health status indexes — in particular we have paid little attention to their use in medical research itself, when concerned with the effectiveness of treatment — they are sufficient to convey the wide applicability of the ideas and techniques we have discussed.

In the remainder of this chapter we discuss the directions that might be taken in Ontario with regard to health status measurement. In particular we examine those areas where it would seem that health status measures may most productively be developed and used and how some of the problems we have discussed in the foregoing, particularly those concerned with questions of value, might be resolved in a practical context.

THE INSTALMENTS TO FOLLOW

There can be little doubt that the contemporary scene concerning health care in both Canada and Ontario is itself healthy. Not only have the principal stages of ensuring easy access to good care been successfully accomplished, but there has been no sitting back on laurels since the enactment of the main legislation at federal and provincial levels. Both federal and provincial governments have shown a keen perception of the value of modern medical care and while they may not always have quite avoided a rather crude reaction to rising expenditure, they have nevertheless both encouraged and participated in a public discussion concerning objectives, ways, and means in the health territory. With increasing movement towards the regionalization of health management in the province, the provincial government has also shown itself able and keen to discuss the most effective ways of implementing it.

In the immediate future there seem to be two principal areas in which health status measures could be used to great advantage. These are, first, as important information to district health councils and, second, as 'output' measures used in specific pieces of research, whether economic, administrative, or clinical. The former is a macro measure, for use in routine decision-making. It also provides an excellent *context* for the latter, micro, measures, by focusing everyone's attention on the central objective of the provincial health services.

It takes very little thought before one realizes, however, that the potential scope of proliferating time-consuming and financially costly surveys is enormous. We need therefore to be discriminating. Of the two broad areas of micro and macro analysis, this scope of proliferation is widest in the micro areas where, conceivably, each study might invent and develop its own health status measure appropriate for the specific problem at hand. We take this first.

At the general level it should be a basic requirement of *all* empirical health research concerned with having impact upon the welfare of patients that due attention be paid to systematic measurement of the outcomes in terms of social functioning. In particular, however, research studies mounted with a view to informing *policy*, should be *required* to assess outcomes. A useful set of criteria has been devised by Williams concerning when the pay-off to such outcome appraisal is likely to be highest:

'among the ingredients ... would be that (i) sizeable amounts of scarce resources are at stake: (ii) responsibility is fragmented; (iii) the objectives of the respective parties are at variance or unclear; (iv) there exist acceptable alternatives of a radically different kind; (v) the technology underlying each alternative is well understood and (vi) the results of the analysis are not wanted in an impossibly short time, items (i), (ii), and (iii) on this list specify situations in which the potential benefits ... would be great, items (iv), (v) and (vi) ensure that the analyst would have something worthwhile to consider.' (Williams, 1974a, 253)

Areas where all these criteria seem to apply in Ontario would especially include policy concerning the balance of community (ambulatory) and institutional care, particularly for the mentally ill and for the elderly. A *locus classicus* for the arguments in favour of treating mental patients in the community (a procedure made possible by developments in psychotropic drugs) is Langsley and Kaplan (1968) and Ontario has not been behind other countries in its 'de-institutionalization' program which has proceeded both far and fast (though neither far nor fast enough for some clinical enthusiasts who, in this instance, find themselves in – unholy – alliance with the philistine cash accounts though not, perhaps, with the economists who are likely to ask more searching questions both about outcome and social cost).

Yet as recently as 1976, Murphy, Englesmann and Tcheng-Laroche in their follow-up study of adult psychotic patients discharged from Canadian hospitals to foster homes were able to comment '... when one examines what is written about the effect of such placement on the patients, one finds much loose description and theory but little hard fact. It has to be said, therefore, that some mental health administrations have been switching quite large numbers of patients into this type of care without any real knowledge of what it is likely to achieve' (p. 179). Amongst their own results, they found that after eighteen months, the decline in symptoms was about the same for the foster home group as for the control group in hospital but that there was no significant improvement (contrary to all expectations) in social 'functioning' as measured by the Katz Community Adjustment Scale (actually a measure not of functioning in general, but of social integration). Much earlier, Herjanic, Hales and Stewart (1969) had found that 25 per cent of those discharged from Saskatchewan Hospital Weyburn were later readmitted, particularly those who were younger patients, who were on high tranquillizer dosages and – significantly enough – those who were closely supervised by the clinic team.

The apparent 'failures' in this de-institutionalization program would be attributed by many to inadequate community resources. Yet what resources are 'adequate'? As White and Hunter (1976) have said in the context of substituting non-MD for MD personnel in community psychiatry, 'our reckoning of cost-effectiveness is ultimately based on measures of life-quality change and what is spent to achieve it ... these indices are notoriously difficult to come by' (p. 19). Yet the paradox remains that the absence of the most crucial piece of information has not stopped a major switch in policy from taking place.

As far as the elderly are concerned, Ontario's very high rate of institutionalization (9.2 per cent in 1972 according to Schwenger 1974, which is about twice the British and American rates) together with the prospect of a relatively rapid growth in members of the over 65s compared with younger age-groups, and bottle-necks in hospitals coupled with vacancies in residential homes, imply that the problems of coping with an ageing population are likely to be at least as difficult in Ontario as elsewhere. Yet in both these cases (the elderly and the mentally sick) there is precious little information about the impact of different kinds of environment (e.g., home care, hostels, and 'half-way houses,' active treatment hospitals, chronic units and hospitals, psychiatric hospitals, nursing homes, etc.) upon the health status (or general well-being) of such patients. Nor is there much information on the true *social* costs (to be distinguished from public expenditure costs) of the alternative regimes of care.

While these two examples of programs cry out for a comprehensive assessment of effectiveness in terms of the health status of patients under alternative regimes, and of the full (social) costliness of the alternatives, it is not our intention to suggest that these areas are the only priority areas for evaluation. *Any* programs that meet the criteria above should be given priority for assessment of this kind. Moreover, it should be a requirement of all research projects that are publicly funded and which purport either to assess clinical effectiveness and/or costliness, that they should develop the outcome measures without which such exercises must remain, at least from a policy view, largely irrelevant (save for the special cases where either effectiveness or costliness is zero).

In all these cases of individual program, activity or procedure assessment, it will be likely that a different outcome measure will be needed. While all should relate to ability to function in society without pain or anxiety, the dimensions of function considered relevant will depend upon both client groups, health problem, and technology: a measure suitable for elderly persons will not usually be suitable for children, nor will a measure suitable for renal failure cases normally be the same as that for head injury victims.

At the present state of development of the art, it does not seem realistic to require that these different measures should be made comparable with one another for the purposes of explicit inter-program evaluation, desirable though this would, on general grounds, be. Rather, their use is seen as being in evaluating alternative ways of doing a specific program. Such evaluation will, however, raise most of the technical and value questions discussed in chapters four and five. The most fundamental of these concerns the dimensions of function to be used, which should be sorted out as explicitly as possible, in terms of the objectives of the program, between those performing the evaluation and their clients (ultimately the Ministry of Health). Explicit attention should then be paid to the trade-offs among these dimensions. In particular, the analysts should ask (a) whether it seems appropriate that the weights should be constant, and (b) whether the scores in each dimension are to be reasonably regarded as separable and additive. If the answer to both these questions is 'yes,' then a simple technique such as that used by Amelia Harris (see chapter five) might be appropriate. If the answer is 'no,' then a technique making pairwise comparisons between *collections of attributes* would be more appropriate, using the 'standard gamble' or 'time trade-off' techniques.

In *every* case, however, two conditions should be insisted upon: (a) the characteristics of those making the value judgments should be identified and the reasons for selecting these judges should be made clear; (b) the sensitivity of the final results to changes in the weights should be tested. With the information this provided, policy makers are in a much better position to form a view of the 'acceptability' of the judgments and also to form a judgment themselves about how crucial some of the value judgments may be in producing the final results.

The extensive potential proliferation of health status measures *in micro studies* is, then, to be expected and, indeed, encouraged. Since, however, such evaluative exercises tend to be one-shot in nature, rather than serving an on-going monitoring purpose, this will not lead to the statistical jungle that might otherwise appear to be looming. Our first specific recommendation is thus that outcome measurement in evaluation projects should be not merely encouraged, but insisted upon. The methods and examples discussed in earlier chapters should provide ample guidance as to how those performing the evaluations might proceed.

The second major priority area for development of health status measures was as planning guides for District Health Councils. This area of development is worthy of a very substantial outlay of public funds. While there is no need here to reiterate the arguments for area measures of health status (see chapters six and seven) the technical questions raised by such an exercise will normally warrant different answers from those of the micro studies, even though the conceptual issues remain largely the same; partly because such an exercise is ongoing; partly because being routinized requires more simplification of procedure than is necessary in specific evaluations; partly because mass surveys also require a similar simplification; and partly because of the desirability of linking such a survey to others, in particular here, to the Canada Health Survey, or to other data sources such as those provided by OHIP.

As we noted earlier, the Ontario Council of Health (1975) has been making some excellent noises about health statistics in the province. It has emphasized the importance of *evaluation* and of data availability on the sub-provincial level of health jurisdictions and program sectors. It has also noted the deficiencies in regard for health status information both for research purposes (especially as they saw it, epidemiological research) and for planning: 'the health statistics system should therefore provide for a continuing survey of health problems, status, needs, and wants ... regularly and at reasonable time intervals ... for use in the planning operation, and evaluation of health services and programs in Ontario' (pp. 18, 21). It also rightly emphasized the importance of *accessibility* of this information: 'the primary users of such information are private individuals, public health professionals, educational institutions, and various community organizations' (30).

The important temptation to resist in an exercise of this sort is to try to obtain too much information not only because this reduces response rates but more especially because it can lead to a sacrifice of information concerning the principal object of the effort: health status. This means, for example, that social functioning in terms of activities of daily living (see chapter five) should be the central emphasis, together with measures of physical and mental discomfort. Measurement of clinical symptoms and days off work are relatively unimportant: the former because they do not describe health status; the latter because they are the consequences of restrictions of activity, not the restrictions themselves, and are much affected by other social characteristics (one-legged professors are professors; one-legged footballers are not footballers).[1] These data should be supplemented by demographic data of the standard type (age, sex, number of dependents, size of family) and by a selective set of other data relating to social characteristics of respondents, which might include, for example, a measure of quality of housing, educational attainment and income, and which are broadly relevant in decisions concerning a choice of institutional or ambulatory care.

Information on utilization should not be sought unless it proves impossible or unethical to make a linkage with OHIP data via the respondents' OHIP numbers. The object of the exercise is not so much to examine utilization as to measure health status through time. Nevertheless, should the OHIP link not be possible, to make available basic information about consultations with GPs and hospital admissions in the recent past would be useful in identifying a broad indication that there may be unmet need.

A link with the Canada Health Survey would also be valuable, possibly by including the questions in that survey concerning functional capacity in the provincial survey.

Unlike the micro measures of health status, which we have discussed above, the value questions concerning choice of dimensions and trade-offs will all have to be made at a central level and considerably less sophistication will be possible here than in the micro measures. In particular, the weights assigned to the chosen measures will probably have to be fixed rather than variable and the sources assigned to functional ability in each dimension will be additive. The British Harris survey provides a model for the kind of procedure that is likely to be most feasible. To avoid 'over-interpretation' of the numerical results they would be best presented (*a*) separately by functional dimensions, and (*b*) *in aggregated form only in ranges*. Such a presentation also maximizes their usefulness to the various users of the information.

It is tempting at this stage to present a list of dimensions of physical functioning, painfulness, and emotional distress, together with the appropriate weights, which should be used in such an exercise. To do so would, however, be quite inappropriate for an 'outsider,' for to do so would be to describe, in as

---

1 Brenda Lundman tells me of the one-legged football player in the Southern US who punts with an artificial leg. So much for the difference between the three English varieties of football and the American!

precise a form as one is ever unlikely to see, the content of Ontario policy. Such a content cannot be merely asserted – either by an 'outsider' or an 'insider' – for it should properly emerge from a dialogue, specifically addressed to the questions we have raised both here and especially in chapter five; a dialogue between the ministry, health professionals, and informed laymen with the advice of experts in both social surveys and the construction of health status measures. Our analysis here should, however, substantially ease their task by having described the issues of principle, by having illustrated how the abstract techniques can be operationalized, and by having identified what appear to be some priority areas to focus upon.

At the present time, conditions augur well for the kind of exercise we have advocated here. Both at the federal and provincial level there has lately been a spate of policy papers whose aims and ideas are close to those serving as the axioms of this book. These have been supplemented (and, of course, preceded) by many papers and monographs emanating from academic, administrative, and semi-official sources which, as can be seen from the many quotations we have taken from them, share the same basic aspirations.

If this book has shown that what is desirable is also possible, then it will have been worthwhile. And if we have been as meticulous as we hope in spotting the pitfalls, and alerting the unwary to step with care, the chances are that an early start can be made with confidence and a high probability of success. The question that has lacked a specific answer outside the specificities of small-scale research projects in health status measurement has, to date, been 'how'? That is the question to which we have attempted to provide the answer and if this final paragraph sounds somewhat like a 'call to arms,' that, of course, is what it frankly is! The question is now 'when do we get down to serious business?'

Bibliography

Ackerknecht, E.W. (1947) 'The role of medical history in medical education.' *Bulletin of the History of Medicine* 21

Aday, L.A. and R. Anderson (1975) *Access to Medical Care* (Ann Arbor: Health Administration Press)

Airth, A.D. and D.J. Newell (1962) *The Demand for Hospital Beds: Results of an Enquiry on Tee-sides* (Newcastle: University of Durham)

Akehurst, R.L. and A.J. Culyer (1975) 'The economic surplus and the value of life.' *Bulletin of Economic Research*

Alchian, A.A. (1953) 'The meaning of utility measurement.' *American Economic Review* March

Algie, J. (1972) 'Evaluation and social service departments.' In W.A. Laing (ed.), *Evaluation in the Health Services* (London: Office of Health Economics)

Allen, R.G.D. (1932) 'The foundations of a mathematical theory of exchange.' *Economica* 12, 197-226

Anderson, O.W. (1972) *Health Care: Can There Be Equity?* (New York: Wiley)

Apple, D. (1960) 'How laymen define illness.' *Journal of Health and Human Behaviour* 1, 219-25

– (ed.) (1960) *Sociological Studies of Health and Sickness* (New York: McGraw-Hill)

Arrow, K.J. (1963) *Social Choice and Individual Values* (2nd ed.) (New York: Wiley)

Baumann, B. (1961) 'Diversities in conceptions of health and physical fitness.' *Journal of Health and Human Behaviour* 2, 39-46

Beaton, G.H. (1976) 'Community health: a new approach in the University of Toronto.' *Canadian Journal of Economics* 9

Beck, R.G. (1973) 'Economic class and access to physicians' services under public medical care insurance.' *International Journal of Health Services*
– (1974) 'The effects of co-payment on the poor.' *Journal of Human Resources* 9
Berg, R.L. (1973) *Health Status Indexes* (Chicago: Hospital Research and Educational Trust)
Blishke, W.R., J.W. Bush and R.M. Kaplan (1975) 'Successive intervals analysis of preference measures in a health status index.' *Health Services Research*, summer
Breton, A. (1974) *The Economic Theory of Representative Government* (London: Macmillan)
Brook, R.H. (1973a), 'Discussion.' In Berg (1973, 38)
– (1973b), *Quality of Care Assessment: A Comparison of Five Methods of Peer Review* (Washington, DC: US Department of Health, Education and Welfare)
Central Statistical Office (CSO) (1975) 'Editorial.' *Social Trends* 6 (London: HMSO)
Chen, M.K. (1973) 'The G index for program priority.' In Berg (1973)
Chinnappa, B.N. (1976) *Notes on the Sample Design for the Canada Health Survey*. Statistics Canada (mimeo)
Coase, R.H. (1960) 'The problem of social cost.' *Journal of Law and Economics* 3
Cochrane, A.L. (1975) 'World health problems.' *Canadian Journal of Public Health* 66, no. 4
Cohen, W.J. (1968) 'Social indicators: statistics for public policy.' *American Statistician* 22, 14-16
Committee on the Healing Arts (1970) *Report* (Toronto: Queen's Printer)
Cooper, M.H. and A.J. Culyer (1972) 'Equality in the NHS: intentions, performance and problems in evaluation.' In M.M. Hauser (ed.), *The Economics of Medical Care* (London: Allen and Unwin)
– and A.J. Culyer (1973) *Health Economics* (London: Penguin)
Culyer, A.J. (1971) 'The nature of the commodity "health care" and its efficient allocation' *Oxford Economic Papers* 23
– (1973) *'Quids* without *quos:* a praxeological approach.' In A.A. Alchian *et al.*, *The Economics of Charity* (London: Institute of Economic Affairs)
– (1974) *Economic Policies and Social Goals: Aspects of Public Choice* (London: Martin Robertson)
– (1976) *Need and the National Health Service* (London: Martin Robertson)
– and J. Cullis (1976) 'Some economics of hospital waiting lists in the NHS.' *Journal of Social Policy* 4
– R.J. Lavers, and A.H. Williams (1971) 'Social indicators: health.' *Social Trends*, no. 2

- J. Wiseman, and A. Walker (1977) *An Annotated Bibliography of Health Economics* (London: Martin Robertson)

Davis, K. and R. Reynolds (1975) 'Medicare and the utilization of health care services by the elderly.' *Journal of Human Resources* 10, 361-77

de Dombal, F.T. *et al.*, (1972) 'Computer-aided diagnosis of acute abdominal pain.' *British Medical Journal* 2, 9-13

Donabedian, A. (1966) 'Evaluating the quality of medical care.' *Milbank Memorial Fund Quarterly* 44 (supplement), 166-207

- (1973) *Aspects of Medical Care Administration: Specifying Requirements for Health Care* (Cambridge, Mass.: Harvard UP)

Economic Council of Canada (1971) *Design for Decision-Making: An Application to Human Resources Policies, ECC Eighth Annual Review* (Ottawa: Information Canada)

- (1974) *Economic Targets and Social Indicators, Eleventh Annual Review* (Ottawa: Information Canada)

- (1975) *Options for Growth, Twelfth Annual Review* (Ottawa: Information Canada

Evans, R.G. (1974) 'Supplier-induced demand: some empirical evidence and implications.' In M. Perlman (ed.), *The Economics of Health and Medical Care* (London: Macmillan)

- (1976) Review of M. Perlman (ed.), *The Economics of Health and Medical Care, Canadian Journal of Economics* 9, 532-7

Fanshel, S. (1972) 'A meaningful measure of health for epidemiology.' *International Journal of Epidemiology* 1, no. 4

- and J.W. Bush (1970) 'A Health-status index and its application to health status outcomes.' *Operations Research*, Nov/Dec

Fraser, R.D. (1972) *The Economics of Health Research*, parts I-VI. (Kingston: Queens University, Institute for Economic Research discussion papers 103-108). Also in Ontario Council of Health (1973)

Friedson, E., (1970), *Profession of Medicine: A Study of the Sociology of Applied Knowledge* (New York: Dodd, Mead and Co.)

Friedsam, H.J. and H.W. Martin (1963) 'A comparison of self and physicians' health ratings in an older population.' *Journal of Health and Human Behaviour* 4, no. 3

Georgescu-Roegen, N., (1952) 'A diagrammatic analysis of complementarity.' *Southern Economic Journal* 19, 1-20

Greenberg, J. (1974a), *Social Indicators in Education: A Conceptual Framework*, Economic Council of Canada discussion paper no. 6 (Ottawa: ECC)

- (1974b) *Social Indicators in Education: A Case Study*, Economic Council of Canada discussion paper no. 15 (Ottawa: ECC)

Grogono, A.W. and D.J. Woodgate (1971) 'Index for measuring health.' *The Lancet* Nov. 6

Grossman, M. (1972) *The Demand for Health: a theoretical and empirical analysis* (New York and London: Columbia University Press)

Gustafson, D.H. and D.C. Holloway (1975) 'A Decision Theory Approach to Measuring Severity in Illness.' *Health Services Research* 10, 97-106

Guttman, L. (1944) 'A basis for scaling qualitative data.' *American Sociological Review* 9

Hardy, J.D., H.G. Wolff, and H. Goodell (1952) *Pain Sensations and Reactions* (Baltimore: Wilkins and Wilkins)

Harris, A., *et al.* (1971), *Handicapped and Impaired in Great Britain* (London: HMSO)

Henderson, D.W. (1974) *Social Indicators: A Rationale and Research Framework* Economic Council of Canada (Ottawa: Information Canada)

Herjanic, M., R.C. Hales, and A. Stewart (1969) 'Does it pay to discharge the chronic patient? A 2 year follow-up of 338 chronic patients.' *Acta Psychiatrica Scandinavica* 45, 53-61

Illich, I. (1975) *Medical Nemesis: The Expropriation of Health* (Toronto: McClelland and Stewart)

Jennett, B. (1974) 'Surgeon of the seventies.' *Journal of the Royal College of Surgeons of Edinburgh* 19, 1-12

Jones-Lee, M. (1976) *The Valuation of Human Life* (London: Martin Robertson)

Katz, S., A.B. Ford, R.W. Maskowitz, B.S. Jackson and M.W. Jaffee (1963) 'The index of ADL: a standardized measure of biological and psychosocial function.' *Journal of the American Medical Association*, Sept. 21

Klarman, H.E. (1965) *The Economics of Health* (New York and London: Columbia University Press)

– (n.d.) 'Socio-economic impact of heart disease.' In *The Heart and Circulation.* Second national conference on cardiovascular diseases (Washington, DC)

– J.O. Francis and G.D. Rosenthal (1968) 'Cost effectiveness applied to the treatment of chronic renal disease.' *Medical Care* 6

Koos, E.L. (1954) *The Health of Regionville* (New York: Columbia)

Lalonde, M. (1974) *A New Perspective on the Health of Canadians* (Ottawa)

Langsley, D.G. and D.M. Kaplan (1968) *The Treatment of Families in Crisis* (New York: Grune and Stratton)

Law, M.M., R. Steele and A.S. Kraus (1973) 'Measuring the impact of a district health unit – a baseline study.' *Canadian Journal of Public Health* 64

Levine, D.S. and D.E. Yett (1973) 'A method for constructing proxy measures of health status.' In Berg (1973)

Lindsay, C.M. (1969) 'Medical care and the economics of sharing.' *Economica* (144)

Lipworth, L., J.H. Lee, and J.N. Morris (1963) 'Case Fatality in teaching and non-teaching hospitals.' *Medical Care* 1

Manga, P. (1976) *A Benefit Incidence Analysis of the Public Medicine and Hospital Insurance Programs in Ontario* Unpublished PhD thesis (University of Toronto)

Maslove, A.M. (1975) '*Indicators and Policy Formation.*' Carleton economic papers no. 6

Maslow, A.H. (1954) *Motivation and Personality* (New York: Harper)

McDowell, I. and C.J.M. Martini (n.d.) *Problems and New Directions in the Evaluation of Primary Care.* (Nottingham University, Department of Community Health)

Mead, M. (1950) *Sex and the Temperament in Three Primitive Societies.* (New York: Mentor)

Mechanic, D. (1968) *Medical Sociology: A Selective View.* (New York: Free Press)

Miller, J.E. (1970) 'An indicator to aid management in assigning program priorities.' *Public Health Reports* 85, no. 8

Murphy, H.B.M., I. Englesmann, and F. Tcheng-Laroche (1976) 'The influence of foster home care on psychiatric patients.' *Articles on General Psychiatry* 33, 179-83

Neumann, J. von, and O. Morgenstern (1953) *The Theory of Games and Economic Behaviour* (3rd ed.) (New York: Wiley)

Office of Health Economics (1964) *New Frontiers in Health* (London: OHE)

Olson, M. (1969) 'The plan and purpose of a social report.' *The Public Interest* no. 15

– (1970) 'An analytic framework for social reporting and policy analysis.' *Annuals of the American Academy of Political and Social Science*, March

Ontario Council of Health (1975) *Health Information and Statistics* (Toronto: Ontario Council of Health)

– (1976) *Evaluation of Primary Health Care Services* (Toronto: Ontario Council of Health)

Ontario Economic Council (1976) *Health: Issues and Alternative* (Toronto: OEC)

Ontario Ministry of Health (1974) *Hospital Statistics 1974* (Toronto: Ministry Information System Division

Organization for Economic Cooperation and Development (1976) *Measuring Social Well-being: A Progress Report on the Development of Social Indicators* (Paris: OECD)

Parsons, T. (1951) *The Social System* (New York: Free Press)
– (1964) *Social Structure and Personality* (New York: Free Press) esp. 258-91
– E. Shils, K.D. Naegele, and J.R. Pitts (eds.) (1961) *Theories of Society* (New York: Free Press of Glencoe)
Patrick, D.L., J.W. Bush, and M.M. Chen (1973) 'Methods for measuring levels of well-being for a health status index.' *Health Services Research* 8, 228-45
Pauly, M.V. (1971) *Medical Care at Public Expense* (New York: Washington, and London: Praeger)
Pearse, I.H. and L.H. Crocker (1949) *The Peckham Experiment* (London: Allen and Unwin)
Piachaud, D. and J.M. Weddel (1972) 'The economics of treating varicose veins *International Journal of Epidemiology* 3
Pole, D. (1971) 'Mass radiography: a cost-benefit approach.' In G. McLachlan (ed.), *Problems and Progress in Medical Care: 5* (Oxford: OUP)
Roemer, M. (1961) 'Bed supply and hospital utilization: a natural experiment.' *Hospitals* 35
Romeder, J.-M. and G.B. Hill (1977) *Priorities and strategies for preventive actions.* Long Range Health Planning Branch Staff Paper 77-4 (Ottawa: Health and Welfare Canada)
Royal Commission on Health Services (1964) *Report* 2 vols (Ottawa: Queen's Printer)
Schwenger, C.W. (1974) 'Keep the old folks at home.' *Canadian Journal of Public Health* 65
Sellin, T. and M.E. Wolfgang (1964) *The Measurement of Delinquency* (New York: Wiley)
Sen, A.K. (1970) *Collective Choice and Social Welfare* (Edinburgh: Oliver and Boyd)
Skinner, D.E. and D.E. Yett (1973) 'Debility index for long-term care patients.' In Berg (1973)
Somers, H.M. and A.R. Somers (1967) *A Program for Research in Health Economics* Health economics series no. 7 (Arlington, Va.: US Department of Health, Education and Welfare, Public Health Service)
Special Program Review (1975) *The Report of the Special Program Review* (Toronto: Ontario Government Bookstore)
Stephens, T.M. (1976) *A Guide to Content Development Prepared by the Canada Health Survey Project Team* (Introduction by T.M. Stephens (Ottawa: Department of National Health and Welfare, mimeo)
Stouman, K. and I.S. Falk (1936) 'Health indices: a study of objective indices of health in relation to environment and sanitation.' *League of Nations Quarterly Bulletin of the Health Organization* 5

Streib, G.F., E.A. Suchman, and B.S. Phillips (1958) 'An analysis of the validity of health questionnaires.' *Social Forces* 36, 223-32

Task Force (1974) *Report of the Health Planning Task Force* (Chairman, J.F. Mustard) (Toronto)

Tenhouten, W.D. (1969) 'Scale Gradient Analysis: a statistical method for constructing and evaluating Guttman scales.' *Sociometry* 32, 80-98

Torrance, G.W. (1970) *A Generalized Cost-effectiveness Model for the Evaluation of Health Programs* (Hamilton: Faculty of Business, McMaster University)

- (1976a) 'Health status indicators: a unified mathematical view.' *Management Sciences* 22, 990-1001

- (1976b) 'Social preferences for health states: an empirical evaluation of three measurement techniques.' *Socioeconomic Planning Sciences* 10, 129-36

- W.H. Thomas, and D.L. Sackett (1972) 'A utility maximization model for evaluation of health care programs.' *Health Services Research* summer

- D.L. Sackett, and W.H. Thomas (1973) 'Utility maximization model for program evaluation: a demonstration application.' In Berg (1973)

Turvey, R. (1963) 'Present value *versus* internal rate of return.' *Economic Journal* 73, no. 289

Twaddle, A.C. (1969) 'Health decisions and sick role variations: an exploration.' *Journal of Health and Social Behaviour* 10, 105-15

Weisbrod, B.A. (1961) *Economics of Public Health*, Philadelphia, University of Pennsylvania Press

- (1971) 'Costs and benefits of medical research: a case study of poliomyelitis.' *Journal of Political Economy* 79, no. 3

White, N.F. and D.G. Hunter (1976) 'Instead of psychiatrists: a critical look at non-medical manpower.' *Canadian Journal of Public Health* 67, 15-20

Williams, Alan (1974a) 'The cost-benefit approach.' *British Medical Bulletin* 30, no. 3

- (1974b) '"Need" as a demand concept (with special reference to health.' In Culyer (1974)

Williamson, J.W. (1971) 'Evaluating quality of patient care: a strategy relating outcome and process assessment.' *Journal of the American Medical Association* 218

Wolfson, A. (1974) *A Health Index for Ontario* (Toronto: Ministry of Treasury and Intergovernmental Affairs)

Wolfson, A. and A. Solari (1976) 'Research report on the results of the patient utilization study.' Ontario Ministry of Labour, Toronto

Ontario Economic Council Research Studies

Lightning Source UK Ltd.
Milton Keynes UK
UKHW010001210722
406167UK00001B/232